A Seven-Step Program
for Getting Through
Menopause
and Enjoying a
Longer, Healthier Life
without drugs

A Seven-Step Program
for Getting Through
Menopause
and Enjoying a
Longer, Healthier Life
without drugs

REVISED EDITION

by

Catherine D. Lowes

HEALTH ISSUES
Toronto, Canada
1998

Published in Toronto, Canada by

Health Issues
P.O. Box 64, Station Q
Toronto, Ontario
Canada
M4T 2L7

Canadian Cataloguing in Publication Data

Lowes, Catherine D., 1950-
    A seven step program for getting through menopause and enjoying a longer, healthier life, without drugs

Rev. ed.
Includes bibliographical references and index.
ISBN 0-9681492-1-9

    1. Menopause—Popular works. 2. Middle aged women—Health and hygiene. I. Title.

RG186.L69 1998   618.1'75   C98-900608-5

Printed and bound in Canada

CONTENTS

INTRODUCTION 1

1 THE CLIMACTERIC & MENOPAUSE 3

Definitions 3

The Pre-Climacteric Menstrual Cycle 4

What Happens During the Climacteric and Menopause? 4

Post-Menopause Hormone Levels 5

Why does Menopause Occur? 6

Why do Women Experience Symptoms? 6

At What Age does Menopause Occur, When it Occurs "Naturally"? 7

When does Menopause Occur "Unnaturally"? 7

Why does the Climacteric Affect so Many Parts of Your Body? 8

Why does the Climacteric Affect each Woman Differently? 8

How do You Know Whether You will have Difficulty? 10

Remember 10

2 SYMPTOMS OF THE CLIMACTERIC 11

Physical Symptoms 12

Emotional Symptoms 17

Intellectual Symptoms 18

Chapter Conclusion 20

Recommended Reading 20

References 20

3 SAYING "NO" TO DRUGS FOR MENOPAUSE 21

Why are Drugs Prescribed to Women during the Climacteric? 21

Drug Groups 22

Conclusion on Drugs 26

Where to Get More Detailed Information on Prescription Drugs 26

4 TRACKING YOUR WAY THROUGH THE CLIMACTERIC 29

Step 1: *Set Up a Menopause Tracking System* 29

Example Calendar 31

Cycle Chart 32

5 ASSESSING THE CURRENT STATE OF YOUR HEALTH 35

Step 2: *Find a Health Practitioner You Trust* 35

Step 3: *Complete the Process of Medical Testing* 35

Why Have Medical Tests? 36

Recommended Medical Tests 36

Test Preparation Information 37

Notes to the Test Checklist 44

Test Checklist 45

The Easy Steps of Examining Your Own Breasts 47

6 UNDERSTANDING YOUR TEST RESULTS 49

Step 4: *Identify Your Health Vulnerabilities* 49

Climacteric/Menopause 50

Cardiovascular 54

Bones 57

References 64

7 GETTING THROUGH THE MENOPAUSAL YEARS 67
WITHOUT DRUGS

Step 5: *Relieve Menopausal Symptoms without Drugs* 68

Herbs 68

Traditional Chinese Medicine 69

Diet 71

Exercise 73

Non-Drug Solutions to Some Difficult Menopausal Symptoms 74

Chapter Conclusion 81

Other Recommended Reading 81

8 IMPROVING YOUR LONG-TERM HEALTH PROSPECTS 83

Step 6: *Start the Process of Changing to a Healthier Diet* 85

Six Goals for a Healthier Diet 86

Step 7: *Enjoy the Benefits of* <u>*Moderate*</u> *Exercise* 104

Chapter Summary 108

References 109

9 OSTEOPOROSIS & BONE FRACTURE 111

What is Osteoporosis? 111

Main Factors Thought to Affect Post-Menopausal Bone Health 112

Manage and Protect Your Bone Health Starting Right Now 116

References 118

10 SEVEN-STEP PROGRAM SUMMARY 121

SELECTED BIBLIOGRAPHY OF BOOKS 123

INDEX 125

MAIL ORDER FORM 135

INTRODUCTION

Menopause is still one of the most misunderstood, misdiagnosed, and inappropriately treated stages in a woman's life. As with other hormonally-driven times (during puberty, prior to menstruation, during pregnancy, and after childbirth), symptoms of menopause are often considered emotional, psychological, stress-related, or imagined.

Few medical doctors know how to identify menopausal symptoms as what they really are — the physiological impact of hormonal imbalances and changes. And few know of non-drug methods for alleviating the short-term symptoms, and reducing the long-term health risks, associated with this major change in a woman's hormonal make-up.

Women must educate themselves because, although menopause is a natural process, many serious consequences can result if the more difficult symptoms are not given early, knowledgeable attention. And many serious side-effects can be caused by the drugs which are routinely prescribed for women at this time in their lives.

The first few chapters of this book provide information about the process and symptoms of menopause, and the drugs commonly recommended by doctors for women in mid-life. The *seven-step program* begins in Chapter 4. It is intended to guide and support you through menopause and beyond.

The information in this book comes from my own experience with menopause, combined with in-depth research along the way. My menopausal years were unnecessarily disruptive, because of lack of understanding and inappropriate treatment by medical doctors, including long-practising general practitioners and specialists, men and women alike.

Thankfully, the difficult years have come to an end for me. I sleep well, feel well, and have lots of energy. My intellectual skills have returned. My emotions are stable. My body is calm. I now have a clear understanding of what I must do to protect my health over the long-term, and I want you to know what I have learned.

Information in this book will help to clarify how menopause is affecting you, and the *seven-step program* will suggest gentle, preventative measures for a smoother passage and a longer, healthier life.

Some of the steps may be easy for you, while others will take considerable time and effort to complete. Take your time. Make the effort. Invest in your health.

Take care of yourself.

Cathie Lowes
September 1998

1
THE CLIMACTERIC
& MENOPAUSE

DEFINITIONS

The following definitions will help you understand the menopausal process.

Menopause: By definition, it is the 3-7 days of your final menstrual period.

This is something that can only be known in retrospect. 12 months must pass without a menstrual period before you can safely say that you are post-menopausal. When this happens, you will know that menopause occurred at the time of that last menstrual period.

Climacteric: An extended period of time during which a woman's hormonal milieu changes from a reproductive to a non-reproductive functional state.

This can be a 2-10 year duration, sometimes starting long before the final menstrual period and carrying on for one or two years after the final menstrual period.

A woman usually experiences the most difficult symptoms during the 2-3 years surrounding the time of her final menstrual period. These years are known as *perimenopause.*

Post–Menopause: The stage of a woman's life which begins after her final menstrual period.

From the above definitions, you can see that when women talk about menopause, they are really talking about the climacteric. Menopause itself is a 3-7 day non-event. When women say they are going through menopause, or "the change of life", they are really going through the climacteric.

In this book, the terms "symptoms of the climacteric" and "menopausal symptoms", or "going through the climacteric" and "going through menopause", will be used interchangeably.

THE PRE-CLIMACTERIC MENSTRUAL CYCLE

Before the years of the climacteric, most women have a steady rise and fall of *estrogen* (the hormone which causes blood to line the womb (uterus) in preparation for egg implantation) and *progesterone* (the hormone which causes blood to be discharged via a menstrual period each month impregnation does not occur). The graph below illustrates a common cyclical pattern, with ovulation occurring around day 14, and menstruation starting around day 28.

THE PRE-CLIMACTERIC MENSTRUAL CYCLE

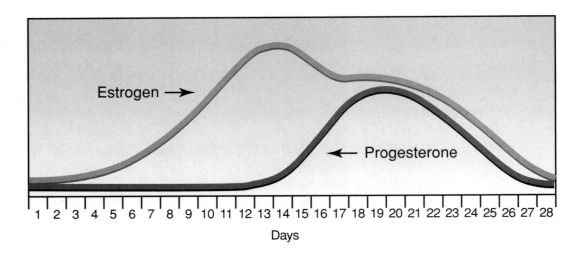

Days

WHAT HAPPENS DURING THE CLIMACTERIC AND MENOPAUSE?

From the beginning of the climacteric to the final menstrual period (menopause), a woman's ovaries go through a process of "winding down" their egg-producing (ovulating) function, as their egg supply diminishes. Menstruation stops when a woman's egg supply is depleted.

Through this "winding down" process, production of estrogen and progesterone fluctuates and declines until those hormones do not fulfill their reproductive functions anymore. They finally settle in at lower, stable, post-menopausal levels.

During the climacteric years, the previously steady ebb and flow of estrogen and progesterone is often replaced by wide swings, more frequent ups and downs, and imbalances between the two hormones.

The following graph illustrates how out of kilter a woman's estrogen and progesterone can get during the climacteric years. Compare the following graph with the common, cyclical pre-climacteric pattern seen above.

In some months (not the one illustrated below), there is insufficient progesterone to cause the blood (uterine lining) to be discharged. These are the months during which a menstrual period does not occur. The next time a menstrual period does occur, a heavier flow may be experienced as more than one month's lining build-up is discharged.

During the climacteric, the length of the menstrual cycle also starts to vary. Minor menstrual cycle changes are usually the first sign that the years of the climacteric have begun.

CLIMACTERIC YEARS

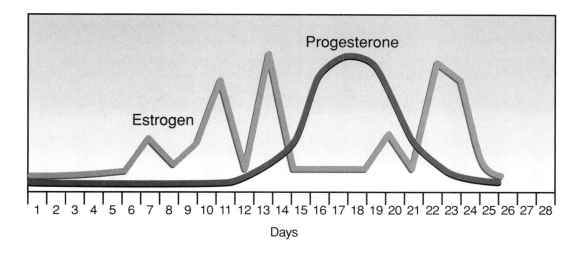

Days

POST-MENOPAUSE HORMONE LEVELS

Once a woman is post-menopausal, estrogen is present in small amounts and remains at a relatively stable level. Progesterone is minimal or absent. This is illustrated in the graph below.

POST-MENOPAUSE

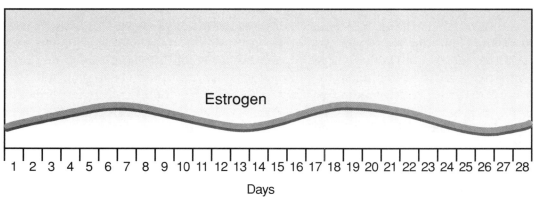

Days

WHY DOES MENOPAUSE OCCUR?

Explanations abound for why menopause occurs. These explanations are, of course, all a matter of opinion and personal theory. The reasons that make the most sense to me are:

1. *Menopause is Nature's way of providing birth control to older women.*

   Pregnancy, giving birth, and raising a child are very physically demanding functions for a woman's body. Both pregnancy and giving birth become higher risk events as a woman's body ages.

2. *Menopause is Nature's way of increasing the chances that a mother will live long enough to nurture her child to adulthood.*

   The mortality rate for mothers is lower in the younger age ranges.

3. *Menopause is Nature's way of reducing deformities in babies.*

   As women grow older, the chance of birth defects increases.

   Just as Nature protects pre-pubertal girls from having babies, by not providing their bodies with the estrogen and progesterone necessary for pregnancy to be possible, Nature also protects older women, by eliminating estrogen and progesterone so that pregnancy cannot occur. In this way, Nature also protects the next generation.

   Estrogen levels are similar in pre-pubertal girls and post-menopausal women. In my opinion, pre-pubertal girls are not estrogen-deficient and *post-menopausal women are not estrogen-deficient*. Both groups have estrogen levels which are appropriate for their reproductive stage of life.

   The post-menopausal years are years when women can be free of the child-bearing role. Because women are living longer today than ever before, this gives them time to experience and enjoy other aspects of life.

WHY DO WOMEN EXPERIENCE SYMPTOMS?

Symptoms occur during the climacteric because of changes and imbalances in a woman's reproductive hormone levels, primarily estrogen, progesterone, and testosterone. Although there is controversy as to which hormone causes the most climacteric-related symptoms, my personal experience has led me to conclude that estrogen is the main symptom-causing culprit. In my opinion, changing levels of estrogen (not the absolute levels, but the fact that the levels are changing), and imbalances between estrogen and progesterone, cause most symptoms of the climacteric.

In the same way that many women experienced tumultuous times in their teenage years when their hormones were "kicking in and out" and working toward settling in at reproductive adult levels, women can experience tumultuous times as their hormones "wind down" to post-reproductive levels. Once a woman's body adjusts to the new, post-menopause hormone levels, symptoms generally stop.

AT WHAT AGE DOES MENOPAUSE OCCUR, WHEN IT OCCURS "NATURALLY"?

("Naturally" means menopause that is not externally induced - see next section)

Menopause is different for every woman, but in general:

- Approximately 1 out of 3 women has her last period by the age of 45.

- Approximately 1 out of 3 women has her last period by the age of 50.

- Approximately 1 out of 3 women has her last period by the age of 55.

From these statistics, you can see how the general public, especially doctors, consider 50 years old to be the magic age for menopause. It is a meaningless and misleading number.

Although 50 may be the approximate *average* age for a woman's final menstrual period, most of the female population experience symptoms of the climacteric long before their 50th birthday. In fact, of those women who have their final menstrual period by the age of 45, many have been experiencing symptoms since their mid-to-late 30s.

A small percentage of women has the last menstrual period after the age of 55.

WHEN DOES MENOPAUSE OCCUR "UNNATURALLY"?

Menopause and symptoms of the climacteric can result from externally induced causes such as:

"Stress Menopause": Menstrual periods can be affected by stress at any time during a woman's life. Serious stress can cause a woman's hormonal milieu to become imbalanced. Job pressures, separation/divorce, bereavement, child-rearing worries, relationship problems, financial difficulties can all cause hormonal imbalances which lead to climacteric-type symptoms.

Hysterectomy: Having your uterus removed can lead to an earlier menopause.

Having your ovaries removed (oophorectomy) always results in immediate menopause due to the abrupt removal of a woman's primary source of estrogen, the ovaries. Women experiencing menopause as the result of an oophorectomy can suffer debilitating symptoms, especially depression. This is a hormonally induced depression, not a psychological depression. It will pass once the body adjusts to its new, lower, hormone levels.

Medical Treatments: Chemotherapy and Radiation can affect ovarian function and cause climacteric-type symptoms. If a woman is close to her time of natural menopause, these treatments may speed up the process and also cause more severe symptoms.

Lupron, a drug used to reduce the size of ovarian cysts and fibroids, by suppressing estrogen production, can cause the onset of climacteric-type symptoms or increase the severity of symptoms already being experienced.

WHY DOES THE CLIMACTERIC AFFECT SO MANY PARTS OF YOUR BODY?

Every important body organ is affected by estrogen and progesterone in some way. There are hormone receptors in hundreds of places in a woman's body - breasts, bones, skin, brain, heart, bowel, bladder, vagina, eyes, etc.

When estrogen and progesterone levels (with which your body has been operating for 30 or so years) change or get out of balance, the function of various body organs is temporarily upset. Once your estrogen and progesterone levels settle in at post-menopausal levels, symptoms generally stop.

WHY DOES THE CLIMACTERIC AFFECT EACH WOMAN DIFFERENTLY?

In my opinion, the climacteric affects each woman differently for five main reasons:

1.   Your body's *sensitivity to hormonal changes* affects how you experience times in your life which are dominated by hormonal changes (e.g., puberty, menstrual periods, pregnancy, after childbirth, the climacteric).

Women experience varying degrees of symptoms and difficulties depending on their sensitivity to their hormonal changes which occur during these times.

2. *Hormonal imbalances* can cause symptoms. Symptoms can result from imbalances in estrogen, progesterone, and testosterone. During puberty, these three hormones establish a relationship with each other which is maintained for decades, through the ups and downs of a woman's monthly cycle. When this relationship changes, symptoms can be experienced.

    A few lucky women never experience hormonal imbalances. Their hormone levels decline slowly and in sync with each other, all the way to the post-menopausal state.

    For many of us, the climacteric includes periods of time when our hormones are out of balance and volatile.

3. *Severity of hormonal changes* differs from woman to woman.

    The *rate* at which hormone levels change, can influence the number and severity of menopausal symptoms.

    A few lucky women glide through the menopausal years, completely unaffected, as their hormone levels taper off gradually and settle at their post-menopausal levels.

    For some unlucky women, hormone levels, especially estrogen, swing wildly up and down, constantly. These are the women whose bodies are in turmoil for several years until the climacteric is over. For these women, symptoms can be so difficult that their ability to function day-to-day can be severely impaired.

    In women for whom menopause occurs due to stress, hysterectomy, or medical treatments, the resulting sharp drop in estrogen can be temporarily devastating.

4. The *impact* of a woman's particular *symptoms on* her specific *life responsibilities* can make the same symptoms almost unnoticeable in one woman and very serious in another. The following examples illustrate the point.

    e.g. A woman with urinary tract sensitivities needs to be close to a washroom because she suffers from urinary frequency and urgency, sometimes for long periods at a time. This symptom would make it difficult for a bus-driver, a travelling saleswoman, or a litigation lawyer to perform her job function.

    e.g. A woman suffering from cognitive dysfunction such as memory loss, difficulty concentrating, and slow thinking would not be able to perform her job as a foreign exchange trader or a bank teller.

    Because menopausal symptoms can last for a number of years, such symptoms can threaten a woman's reputation and livelihood.

5. *Diet* can have an impact on level of suffering. Women who consume foods such as legumes (beans) and soy products, regularly, may experience milder symptoms of the climacteric; whereas, excessive consumption of fat, sugar, caffeine, and foods of animal origin (i.e., meat, fish, fowl, dairy, eggs) is thought to worsen menopausal symptoms.

Chapter 7, "Getting Through the Menopausal Years Without Drugs", lists some of the foods which are considered to be effective in reducing the severity of menopausal symptoms.

HOW DO YOU KNOW WHETHER YOU WILL HAVE DIFFICULTY?

In general:

•   If you have never had hormone-related problems in the past (i.e., not suffered from PMS, or experienced hormone-associated pregnancy or post-partum difficulties), you will be unlikely to have problems with menopause.

•   If you have been sensitive to hormone changes in the past (i.e., suffered from PMS, or experienced hormone-associated pregnancy or post-partum difficulties), you are more likely to experience difficulties with the hormonal changes involved in menopause.

•   If you have been sensitive to hormone changes in the past and/or you are under a lot of stress, or have had a hysterectomy or medical treatments which affect hormones (as outlined earlier), you may experience difficult symptoms.

Suggestions for reducing the severity of menopausal symptoms are provided in Chapter 7, "Getting Through the Menopausal Years Without Drugs".

REMEMBER

In my opinion, the degree of menopausal suffering which any woman experiences is not related to her attitude, her level of physical fitness, or her psychological state.

Women who experience difficulties should never be made to think of themselves as weaklings or failures. Such women need support and encouragement. The difficult times will come to an end once their hormones stabilize at post-menopausal levels.

2
SYMPTOMS OF
THE CLIMACTERIC

This chapter provides an extensive list of symptoms experienced by women going through the climacteric (menopause). No one can claim to know all the ways in which hormonal changes and imbalances affect a woman's body. Most women will experience some, but not all, of the following symptoms. You may experience some that are not included here.

Many of the symptoms described here are not acknowledged by "Western" medical doctors as symptoms of menopause. Most of these symptoms are generally considered to be either a normal part of aging (for both men and women), or caused by something else (e.g., stress, overwork, or an illness).

Indeed, for some women, such symptoms may be caused by stress, overwork, or an illness. To rule out illness, consult your doctor and follow the steps in Chapter 5, "Assessing the Current State of Your Health".

As for the symptoms being a normal part of aging; in my opinion, what differentiates menopausal symptoms from aging is their more severe, but temporary, nature during the climacteric years. My own unique experience leads me to the conclusion that the symptoms outlined in this chapter can be caused by the hormonal changes and imbalances which occur during those years. Here is my story...

My Own Unique Experience

In January, 1994, I was dangerously anemic as the result of months of continuous heavy bleeding; *and* my gynecologist discovered a small cyst on one of my ovaries. In order to stop the bleeding and reduce the size of the cyst, he injected me with the first of three monthly shots of a drug called Lupron.

Lupron had the effect of immediately reducing my body's estrogen to post-menopausal levels. Within two hours of the first injection, I began to experience, very severely, the symptoms outlined in this chapter. Although the drug was supposed to work its way out of my body within the two to four weeks after each injection, my hormones never voluntarily snapped back to their normal state (as evidenced by symptoms and hormone blood tests).

I suffered debilitating symptoms until October, 1994, at which time I was fortunate to find a traditional Chinese doctor who immediately diagnosed the underlying cause of my suffering as hormonal. Dong Quai (a common herbal treatment in the Orient for menopausal symptoms, refer to Chapter 7) was prescribed, and within two weeks of beginning treatment, my symptoms were gone and I was in control of my mind and body again.

I worked my way off Dong Quai over the ensuing four months, and experienced the same, but less severe, symptoms with each dosage reduction. Subsequent to that, I experienced about three years of milder, manageable, symptoms.

The pharmaceutical company, which produces Lupron, listed substantially all of the symptoms in this chapter as adverse reactions documented in two clinical studies of the drug. These include hot flashes, breast tenderness, depression, anxiety, blurred vision, ophthalmologic (eye) disorders, dizziness/light-headedness, headache, hearing disorders, sleep disorders, lethargy, memory loss, mood swings, nervousness, numbness, itching, urinary tract infection, incontinence, frequency/urgency/pain in urination, loss of strength, bone pain, difficulty breathing, and more. These are the identified side-effects of a drug which causes a sharp reduction in estrogen levels in women.[1]

Symptoms of the climacteric have been divided into three categories below: Physical, Emotional, Intellectual.

PHYSICAL SYMPTOMS

Changes in Menstrual Periods

Change in menstrual pattern is one of the first indications that a woman has entered the climacteric (menopausal) years.

Most women experience changes in their menstrual cycle long before other symptoms are noticed. Menstrual periods can change in the following ways:

a) *Menstrual cycles become irregular.* The time between menstrual periods may shorten, lengthen, or generally vary. There may be 28 days between menstrual periods, or 12, 22, 32, 55, etc. Regular periods may occur for a few months, followed by irregularity. Menstrual periods may be missed for months at a time. Nothing is predictable.

b) *Menstrual flow and duration vary.* Some menstrual periods may produce heavy bleeding (flooding), gushing, clotting, which requires tampons, combined with layers of overnight pads, during the day and night. This may last for one to two weeks, or longer, and may eventually lead to iron-deficiency anemia, due to excessive loss of blood.

Some menstrual periods may consist of only a few days of light spotting. Mid-cycle spotting can also occur. Nothing is predictable.

c) *Menstrual colour may change.*

d) *Menstrual cramping may worsen.*

Fatigue

Total exhaustion for days, weeks, or months at a time can be caused by changing hormone levels during the menopausal years. (Remember how tired you were during the first three months of pregnancy?)

Fatigue can also result from lack of sleep due to night sweats or sleep disturbances (see below).

Iron-deficiency anemia, due to heavy menstrual bleeding, can cause fatigue.

Hot Flashes

80% of menopausal North American women experience hot flashes, but they come in so many different forms that they may not be recognized as hot flashes. Hot flashes are often preceded by a "feeling" that something is about to happen.

Here are some of the main ways hot flashes are experienced, but remember, anything goes.

a) A mild rush of warmth starts on the chest and moves upward to the neck and face. It can cause a blotchy or a smooth redness on the skin. Perspiration may form on the skin. The heart may start to race. A chill may follow (mild version).

b) You may feel a rush of heat from the waist up which causes you to become drenched with perspiration. Your heart races. You feel temporarily exhausted, even faint, and have a desperate need to remove clothing or to find a cold place to offset the internal heat. You will require a change of clothes. Chills follow (extreme version).

c) A wave of any of nausea, dizziness, diarrhea, fatigue, heat, and weepiness may come over your body. You may interpret this as a mild virus or a low-grade fever (except that a mild virus doesn't come with weepiness). Chills and shakiness may follow.

Some hot flashes are accompanied by panic attacks, feelings of anxiety or terror, and heart palpitations. Hot flashes are harmless. They can last a couple of minutes (usually) or more than an hour (rarely). They can occur seldom or often, regularly or irregularly. They can occur before and/or after your final menstrual period.

Night Sweats

These are the night-time version of a hot flash.

You may wake up in the middle of the night feeling uncomfortable, and with perspiration on your chest, forehead, or nape of the neck. Chills follow.

You may wake up in the middle of the night with your heart racing and your upper body soaking. Sheets and night clothes may be wet. Chills follow.

You may wake up in the middle of the night with your heart racing and a temporary fever; feeling sick, hot, dizzy, or wet from perspiration; and needing to urinate. Again, you may think you have a virus. Chills follow.

Sleep Disturbances/Insomnia

You may have difficulty falling asleep. Once asleep, you may wake frequently during the night due to night sweats, a disturbing dream, a need to urinate, or no apparent reason.

You may fall asleep easily, but wake up very early in the morning (e.g., 3.a.m.), and not be able to get back to sleep.

Some women have bouts of "sleep apnoea" during which they wake up at night gasping for air due to temporary cessation of breathing.

Air Hunger

During your waking hours you may experience bouts of feeling as if you cannot get enough oxygen or take a deep breath.

Digestive Upset/Discomfort/Bloating

Gastrointestinal changes such as looser bowels, constipation, gas, and indigestion can occur during the menopausal years. Some women develop a sensitivity to wheat and suffer from gas and bloating.

Abdominal bloating may come and go. It may occur for hours at a time, at any time, or it may occur around the time of menstruation. Water retention and bloating are common during the menopausal years, as they are pre-menstrually and during pregnancy.

Pulsating aches that feel like muscle spasms can occur in the lower right or left abdomen and may be accompanied by anxiety and weepiness.

Nausea

Nausea can occur as part of a hot flash or a night sweat. Episodes of nausea, accompanied by diarrhea, fatigue, hyperventilation, warm body temperature, and weepiness may occur. This may feel like a mild virus.

Dizziness

Dizziness can occur with hot flashes, with night sweats, or all alone.

Headaches

Some women experience headaches, including migraines with auras, for the first time, or at a more severe level, during the years of the climacteric. For others, this is the time when years of headaches come to an end.

Head Shocks

Little "zingers" like electrical charges to the head can occur and cause dizziness, agitation, and shakiness. These can result in temporary loss of concentration and memory of what you were just doing. These are often followed immediately by panic attacks, including heart palpitations, and perhaps weepiness.

Heart Palpitations

Your heart may start to beat quickly. This often occurs during hot flashes and night sweats, but can also happen during a time of complete relaxation or just after lying down to go to sleep.

Urinary Problems

Urinary distress can come and go throughout the menopausal years and can be experienced in several different ways. You may experience none or all of the following problems.

a)   urinary frequency - the need to urinate often

b)   "stress incontinence" - leaking a bit of urine when laughing, coughing, sneezing, jumping, running, even walking.

c)   "urge incontinence" - the sudden need to urinate and an inability to hold on long enough to make it to a washroom

d)   bladder infections - more frequently

It is important to find a doctor who can correctly diagnose which one of these conditions you may have. Only infections respond to antibiotics. *Do not take antibiotics unnecessarily.*

Vaginal Problems

Vaginal dryness may occur and result in painful intercourse; vaginal yeast and bacterial infections can increase in frequency; itchiness may occur in the area of the vulva and the vagina; stronger vaginal odours can occur at times.

Joint Pain

Aches, pains, and inflammation in joints anywhere in the body can occur during the menopausal years. This is known as "Menopause Arthritis", because it goes away after the final menstrual period.

The right side of the body seems to be the most frequently affected. Hip pain, shoulder pain, wrist pain, and pain in hands (especially the right hand middle finger) and feet (heels, bunions) are common. The hinged joint of the jawbone can also be affected and sometimes refer pain up to the ear.

Muscles

Muscles may go through periods of being weaker and more wobbly, or rubbery. Reflexes may be slower. Co-ordination may seem impaired.

Muscles may cramp more often, especially in legs and feet. This may waken you in the night.

Lower backache may come and go. This may be more pronounced pre-menstrually.

Skin Sensitivities

"Formication" is a tingly or itchy sensation sometimes felt on the skin, as if bugs are crawling on it.

Sometimes a prickling, burning, or a numb sensation is felt on the skin.

Sensory Disturbances

Vision disturbances are common. You may feel that you cannot focus your eyes, or that your vision has deteriorated, although an eye test does not indicate this. Sharpness of objects may be decreased. Fuzzy vision or spots may occur before the eyes. Dry eyes and periodic eye pain can occur.

Ears may become plugged. They may pop and plug up again, giving a feeling of not being able to hear clearly. Ringing, buzzing, and bursts of sound are common ear disturbances during the menopausal years.

You may feel a dry or burning sensation in your mouth. You may develop bad breath or a bad taste in your mouth. Your tastes may change.

Breast Discomfort

Breast tenderness similar to pre-menstrual or pregnancy breast tenderness is common during the years of the climacteric. This condition can come and go within the menstrual cycle. Breasts can feel so full or hard that they are sore and very painful to touch.

Nipples can become very sensitive and sore to touch.

Weight Gain

A 10 pound weight gain during the menopausal years is not uncommon.

PMS

Can become worse and may last longer.

Fibroids/Ovarian Cysts

Previously harmless fibroids and cysts can grow and cause pain and discomfort during this time of hormonal imbalance.

Changes affecting your Sex Life

Vaginal dryness can cause painful intercourse, or a burning feeling during intercourse, and even for a while afterwards.

Intensity and/or duration of orgasm can reduce somewhat or, orgasm might not be as easy to reach.

Decreased desire for sex in some but not all cases.

EMOTIONAL SYMPTOMS

None of these symptoms are truly "emotional". They are caused by hormonal changes and imbalances. They do not reflect real emotions. They are outside a woman's control and, based on my personal experience, they eventually go away.

Depression/Sadness

Hormonal changes can cause feelings of sadness or melancholy, even serious depression.

You may feel a little "low", or be so depressed that you cannot even get out of bed in the morning. Motivation to perform the simplest and most basic everyday functions, or to participate in the easiest of everyday activities, may disappear.

A different kind of depression can also be caused by discouragement and anger at feeling ill, out of control of your body, and at the mercy of your hormones, for too long.

A woman's self-image, job performance, and personal relationships can be threatened by debilitating menopausal symptoms. The helplessness and frustration, associated with feeling that your life is outside your control, can be very depressing.

Anxiety

Nervousness for long periods of time and a sensation of trembling can also occur. You may fret about more things and feel weak and vulnerable.

Panic Attacks

You may have a sudden feeling of terror or impending doom. Your heart may start to race, your breathing may become quick and shallow. This can occur as part of a hot flash, a night sweat, or alone. It usually lasts a few minutes and is harmless.

Mood Swings

Extremes of emotion are common during the years of the climacteric. Feeling elated and "pumped" one day, may be replaced by feeling depressed and "beaten" the next.

Fearful/Insecure/Vulnerable

Some women go through periods of feeling weak, and fearful of the future. They worry about what tomorrow may bring and how they will cope. Everyday events and responsibilities, previously simple to handle, can seem overwhelming when hormones are out of sync.

Fearfulness can be worsened by the day-to-day reality of struggling to meet responsibilities with impaired abilities, especially if the impaired abilities are crucial to fulfilling such roles as "putting food on the table", or raising children.

Irritable/Angry/Impatient

Some women become uncharacteristically angry, short-tempered, or impatient during the menopausal years. They may pick fights, become confrontational, or generally behave atypically.

Uncharacteristic Crying

Weepiness is common during the menopausal years, just as it is during other times dominated by hormonal changes (e.g., puberty, pre-menstrual days, pregnancy, after child-birth).

The smallest frustration may prove overwhelming and lead to uncharacteristic tearfulness.

A hot flash may bring on a feeling of weepiness, possibly accompanied by nausea and dizziness.

Feeling Crazy/Out of Control

For some women, hormonal changes affect them in ways that are so contrary to their normal selves that they feel, and are, out of control of their bodies.

INTELLECTUAL SYMPTOMS

These are the symptoms which had the greatest impact on my ability to fulfill my responsibilities in life. They were most pronounced during the 5-7 days prior to a menstrual period. Although they were difficult, frightening, and not of brief duration, they are now gone.

Memory Loss

Forgetfulness and absent-mindedness are common during the years of the climacteric. Loss of short-term memory can result in an inability to remember what was said, just moments ago. This may be serious if coupled with a reduced ability to concentrate and focus. Depending on the severity of your symptoms, you may experience difficulty following verbal instructions, completing tasks, or even participating intelligently in a conversation.

Trouble Concentrating/Walking Around in a Fog

There may be times when you cannot focus, or even follow conversations. You may find yourself in situations in which you know your body is there, but your surroundings seem unreal, as if you are looking out from behind a curtain. Some women also experience this during pregnancy.

Difficulty Making Decisions

Some women go through periods of feeling less intellectually "sharp". Because of this, they may be uncomfortable with the quality of their decisions, and anxious about their ability to cope with any consequences. Even the simplest decisions may be difficult to make.

Fuzzy Thinking/Less Mentally Sharp

Although IQ is not affected, you may experience reduced intellectual functioning. It may take longer to absorb or understand new information. It may take longer to find solutions to problems. You may not feel as smart or think as quickly. It may be difficult to work with numbers.

Less able to Organize

You may feel that your circuits are overloaded and that you cannot organize your thoughts or deal with more than one task at a time.

CHAPTER CONCLUSION

Some women suffer very serious and debilitating symptoms of the climacteric, which threaten their personal relationships and financial security. Others are more fortunate and experience varying, but milder, degrees of discomfort. Either way, for most women, the transitional years of the climacteric do not usually last for more than 2-3 years.

It is important to recognize that your symptoms are caused by *temporary* hormonal changes, and to know that your old self will eventually resurface with more depth, strength, and energy than ever before. As much as is practical, involve the people who care about you, in this process of transition. Allow them to provide the support you need.

RECOMMENDED READING

Title:	*the pause*
Author:	Lonnie Barbach
Published:	1994
Publisher:	Penguin Books
ISBN:	0-451-18035-6

References

1. Canadian Pharmacists Association. *Compendium of Pharmaceuticals and Specialties*. Ottawa, Canada: Canadian Pharmacists Association, 1998, pages 918-919.

3
SAYING "NO" TO DRUGS FOR MENOPAUSE

There are numerous ways to reduce the severity of symptoms of the climacteric, and the longer term risks of cardiovascular disease and osteoporosis. The main remedies are: drugs, herbs, traditional Chinese medicine, diet, and exercise.

One of the purposes of this book is to encourage and support women who cannot, or choose not to, use drug remedies. When drugs are used to eliminate one health problem, other problems are often created.

WHY ARE DRUGS PRESCRIBED TO WOMEN DURING THE CLIMACTERIC?

If your health care professional has "Western" medical training, it is likely that you will be given drug prescriptions at some point during the years of your climacteric. In my opinion, these prescriptions will probably be given for the following reasons:

1. *To inappropriately treat climacteric symptoms which have been misdiagnosed as something else*

2. *To treat climacteric symptoms which have been correctly diagnosed*

3. *As standard procedure for a woman approaching menopause*

With drugs, the cure can be worse than the "disease", and the possible side-effects can range from being troublesome to life-threatening. (Although menopause is not a disease, it is often treated as such by doctors.)

In my experience, "Western" doctors tend to down-play the negative side-effects of drugs. This is probably due to their formal training and the influence of drug company promotions. Be careful not to allow your doctor's attitude, or lack of knowledge, to affect *your* decisions about *your* health care. Drugs can damage the body's vital organs and disrupt the body's natural chemical balance.

The next section will provide medical facts about the three drug types most commonly prescribed by doctors for women going through menopause. The possible side-effects listed are not necessarily all the side-effects which can occur. You may experience all, some, or none of them. Everyone's body responds differently to drugs; and, because of the complexity of the human body, full knowledge of the side-effects of any drug, especially over the long-term, can never be known.

Drug information in this book has been obtained primarily from:

Title:	***Complete Guide to Prescription & Non-Prescription Drugs***
Author:	H. Winter Griffith, M.D.
Published:	1997
Publisher:	The Berkley Publishing Group
ISBN:	0-399-52345-6

DRUG GROUPS

Tranquilizers

Tranquilizers reduce anxiety and excitement levels. They are used to induce sleep or relaxation. They affect the part of the brain that controls emotions.

Tranquilizers are not appropriate for anxiety caused by hormonal changes. They treat a symptom without addressing the underlying cause.

There are dozens of different brands of tranquilizers. A couple you may know are:

VALIUM   LORAZEPAM

a) *Possible side-effects of tranquilizers - immediate*

- ADDICTION. (Within about 3 weeks, depending on dosage and frequency. Check with pharmacist.)

- Clumsiness, drowsiness, dizziness

- Confusion, vision changes, depression, hallucinations, fever, chills, dry mouth, irritability, constipation, diarrhea, nausea, vomiting, abdominal pain, difficult urination, headache, behaviour changes

- Impaired intellectual function

b) *Possible side-effects of tranquilizers - prolonged use*

- Can cause liver function impairment

Anti-depressants

Anti-depressants treat mental depression. Different types impact the brain differently.

Anti-depressants are not appropriate for depression caused by hormonal changes. They treat a symptom without addressing the underlying cause.

There are many different brands of anti-depressants. A couple you may know are:

PROZAC   ELAVIL

a) *Possible side-effects of anti-depressants - immediate*

- Tremor, headache, dry mouth or unpleasant taste, constipation, diarrhea, nausea, indigestion, fatigue, weakness, drowsiness, nervousness, anxiety, excessive sweating, insomnia

- Hallucinations, nightmares, blurred vision, eye pain, vomiting, irregular heartbeat, abdominal pain, joint pain, heart palpitations, difficult or frequent urination, painful menstruation, nasal congestion, back pain

- Possible withdrawal symptoms of convulsions, muscle cramps, nightmares, insomnia, and abdominal pain

b) *Possible side-effects of anti-depressants - prolonged use*

- UNKNOWN!

Hormones - Hormone Replacement Therapy (HRT)

Hormone replacement therapy, or HRT for short, means a combination drug regimen to replace the body's natural estrogen and progesterone, which decline throughout the climacteric to lower, post-menopausal levels. The purpose of the drugs is to maintain the higher pre-menopausal estrogen and progesterone levels in a woman's body. The drug form of progesterone is called progestin.

These drugs come in many different forms (e.g., tablet, capsule, patch, cream, suppositories, injection), and under many different brand names (e.g., Premarin, Estraderm for estrogen; Provera for progestin).

a) *Health Benefits of HRT - immediate - (within 3 months)*

- Relieves hot flashes (usually), heart palpitations, dizziness, numbness

- Relieves vaginal dryness, urinary tract infections, stress incontinence

- Ends mood swings, irritability, depression

b) Health Benefits of HRT - prolonged use:

- Thought to protect against cardiovascular disease

- Shown to protect against accelerated bone loss which sometimes occurs in the five or so years following menopause (Author's note: Post-menopausal bone loss does not necessarily occur in all women. Nor does bone loss necessarily lead to broken bones. Refer to Chapter 9, "Osteoporosis & Bone Fracture".)

c) Possible side-effects of estrogen - immediate

- Stomach cramps, appetite loss, nausea, diarrhea, swollen feet and ankles, tender swollen breasts, acne, intolerance of contact lenses, change in menstruation

- Rash, stomach or side pain, bloody skin blisters, breast lumps

- Depression, dizziness, migraine headache, irritability, vomiting

- Hair loss, vaginal discharge or bleeding, changes in sex drive

- In rare instances can cause blood clot in lung, leg, or brain

d) Possible side-effects of estrogen - prolonged use

- Increased risk of gallstones

- Increased growth in uterine fibroids and ovarian cysts

- Increased risk of uterine cancer and breast cancer

e) Possible side-effects of progestin - immediate

- Blood clot in lung, leg, or brain

- Hives, rash, intense itching, faintness soon after a dose

- Appetite or weight changes, swollen feet or ankles, unusual tiredness or weakness, menstrual cycle changes, acne

- Prolonged vaginal bleeding, pain in calf

- Depression, insomnia

- Nausea, tender breasts, headache

- Rash, stomach or side pain, jaundice, fever, vision changes

- May reduce protective benefit which estrogen is thought to provide against cardiovascular disease

f) Possible side-effects of progestin - prolonged use

- UNKNOWN!

The most compelling reason doctors give to persuade women to go on HRT is the claim that it protects against osteoporosis and cardiovascular disease. But HRT does not guarantee protection against osteoporosis or cardiovascular disease; and reduced risk of both diseases can be effected through other means, such as diet, exercise, lifestyle, natural supplementation, and/or non-hormonal drugs specific to osteoporosis or cardiovascular disease.

Dr. Susan Love, renowned breast cancer surgeon, researcher and Director of the Revlon/UCLA Breast Center in Los Angeles, California, reviews the major studies, claims, and theories surrounding HRT in her book:

Title:	***Dr. Susan Love's Breast Book***
Author:	Susan M. Love, M.D.
	with Karen Lindsay
Published:	1995 2nd Edition
Publisher:	Addison-Wesley Publishing Company
ISBN:	0-201-40835-X

In Dr. Love's opinion, and in my opinion, the bottom line on HRT is that the health advantages of taking HRT have not been irrefutably proven, nor are the risks fully understood. On the other hand, diet, exercise, and lifestyle are known to reduce the risks of cardiovascular disease and osteoporosis. All women owe it to themselves to consider the alternatives to hormone drugs.

If your doctor trivializes the risks of HRT, or demonstrates a lack of knowledge of the risks, *find another doctor.* He or she has either not taken the time to thoughtfully study the findings, has been swayed by drug company marketing campaigns, or doesn't care about your long-term health. Whatever the reason, it reflects a perilous attitude and means that your health care is not in *competent hands.*

CONCLUSION ON DRUGS

Going back over the possible negative side-effects of all three drug types, and considering the fact that there are non-drug ways to deal with menopause-related health issues, it is appalling and outrageous that so many doctors prescribe these drugs to so many women.

Women should be seeking out, and incorporating into their lives, non-drug ways to alleviate the short-term symptoms of the menopausal years and to reduce the long-term health risks associated with lower post-menopausal hormone levels.

Chapter 7, "Getting Through the Menopausal Years Without Drugs", provides information which will help you find, and safely use, non-drug methods to reduce the severity of your menopausal symptoms.

Chapter 8, "Improving Your Long-Term Health Prospects", outlines an approach to establishing a diet and lifestyle which will lessen your short-term symptoms of menopause; reduce the long-term health risks associated with lower post-menopausal hormone levels; improve all aspects of your health; and increase your prospects for a long and healthy life.

WHERE TO GET MORE DETAILED INFORMATION ON PRESCRIPTION DRUGS

All the possible side-effects of a drug are seldom known by the prescribing doctor. Nor does the brief information slip, provided by some pharmacists, give the whole story. Before taking any drug, it is wise to fully understand both the short and long-term implications for your health, as identified by the drug company during clinical trials. But remember, the long-term has not occurred yet for many drugs, and the long-term side-effects will only be known when people taking these drugs today, suffer the side-effects later in life.

Detailed information about any prescription drug can be obtained from your pharmacist or at your local library. In Canada, look for the specific drug write-up in the *Compendium of Pharmaceuticals and Specialties* (CPS), put out by the Canadian Pharmacists Association.

In the United States, the equivalent reference is the *U.S. Pharmacopoeia Drug Information* (USPDI), put out by the U.S. Pharmacopoeia Convention.

A SEVEN-STEP PROGRAM

From here forward, this book is set up to provide you with a step-by-step program for getting through menopause and enjoying a longer, healthier life without drugs. The seven steps are found within the chapters which follow, along with detailed information to help you accomplish each one. The seven steps are:

STEP 1
Set Up a Menopause Tracking System.

STEP 2
Find a Health Practitioner You Trust.

STEP 3
Complete the Process of Medical Testing.

STEP 4
Identify Your Health Vulnerabilities.

STEP 5
Relieve Menopausal Symptoms without Drugs.

STEP 6
Start the Process of Changing to a Healthier Diet.

STEP 7
Enjoy the Benefits of Moderate Exercise.

**Take your time. Make the effort.
It is important to your health and to your future.**

4
TRACKING YOUR WAY THROUGH THE CLIMACTERIC

STEP 1: *Set Up a Menopause Tracking System.*

It is valuable to set up a system to track your way through the menopausal years. Record-keeping will serve the following purposes:

- It will become clear, through changes in menstrual periods, that you *are* going through menopause.

- It will reduce fear and uncertainty about the cause of symptoms.

- It will provide information for your doctor to correctly diagnose and appropriately care for you.

This tracking system has three parts. The first two are simple. The third is critical to your long-term health and will be dealt with in its own chapter, following this one.

Part 1: Track your symptoms daily on a calender.

On an 8½" x 11" calendar, like the Example Calendar at the end of this chapter, enter information about symptoms you experience, if any, on a daily basis. Follow the example or do what works for you. As time goes by, symptom patterns will appear, cycle to cycle, or just coming and going between cycles, reflecting hormonal changes.

Once you are familiar with your own pattern of symptoms, you will be reassured that they are hormone-related, and therefore, mostly temporary.

Part 2: Track your menstrual cycles.

Use the Cycle Chart at the end of this chapter to note the number of days between menstrual periods, the duration of each menstrual period, and the amount, colour, and density of your menstrual flow.

As time goes by, a trend will appear. Increased irregularity in any of the above factors is common during the menopausal years. In the last year or two before the final menstrual period, many women will be able to watch their menstrual cycles wind down and come to an end.

You may wish to photocopy the second page of the Cycle Chart a few times before filling it in, and use those blank pages for recording future months' menstrual cycle information.

Part 3: Track your hormone levels, bone density, heart, and health through medical tests.

Chapter 5, "Assessing the Current State of Your Health", provides a program for monitoring your health through the climacteric and beyond, and becoming aware of your personal health vulnerabilities.

Your record-keeping could continue for a number of years, depending on how long your symptoms last or how long you wish to continue recording information.

As you near the end of your menopausal years (the climacteric), you will find your records insightful. Until then, they will provide constant reinforcement for your diagnosis, and take the mystery and fear out of your symptoms.

EXAMPLE CALENDAR

September

Sunday	Monday	Tuesday	Wednesday	Thursday	Friday	Saturday
	1 Day 18 of cycle. Lower right backache & a little tired.	**2** Day 19. No sleep problems. Lots of energy. Most days ears are plugged, popping and ringing.	**3** Day 20. Same as yesterday.	**4** Day 21. 6 p.m. head fogged up, dizzy, weird. Abdominal discomfort. Weepy, confused.	**5** Day 22. Mildly fogged up eyes and ears. Brains OK.	**6** Day 23. Feeling unwell today. Lower right backache.
(7) Day 24- spotting - Feel worse. Periods of feeling warm and ill. Backache worse. Urinary sensitivity.	**(8)** Day 25- spotting - Terrible backache, hip pain. Cold, shaky, felt ill all a.m. Went away around 1 p.m.	**(9)** Day 1- period. Slept OK. Period started in a.m. Spasms in left lower abdomen.	**(10)** Day 2-period. Lower left abdomen pulsating spasms every 30 secs all day. Feel ill & weepy.	**(11)** Day 3- spotting - Pulsating gone. Shaky, cold, waves of feeling like crying. Not much done today.	**(12)** Day 4- spotting. Better today. Only ear and eye problems.	**13** Day 5. Same as yesterday.
14 Day 6. Feel fine in all ways except the usual eyes, ears, head fog.	**15** Day 7. Same as yesterday.	**16** Day 8. Dizzy, difficult time for a few hours in a.m.	**17** Day 9. OK.	**18** Day 10. Restless sleep. Foggy head all day. Memory no good. Weepy & depressed at dinner.	**19** Day 11. Feeling good except eyes, ears. Head working well.	**20** Day 12. Same as yesterday.
21 Day 13. Same as yesterday.	**22** Day 14. Same as yesterday.	**23** Day 15. Same as yesterday.	**24** Day 16. Same as yesterday.	**25** Day 17. Same as yesterday.	**26** Day 18. Same as yesterday.	**27** Day 19. Didn't sleep much last night. Head foggy during day. Breasts & abdomen full.
28 Day 20. Same as yesterday.	**29** Day 21. Same as yesterday.	**30** Day 22. Same as yesterday.				

CYCLE CHART

Date of 1st day of menstrual period	# of days since 1st day of last period	# of days period duration	Nature of menstrual flow (amount, colour, density)
Mar.26/96	43	5	*Day 1:* Started 11 p.m. No pre-spotting. No clotting.
			Day 2: Steady, deep red flow. 4 regular pads in 24 hrs.
			Day 3: Flow slowing. 1 maxi all day would have done.
			Day 4: Less flow. No clots. 1 regular pad all day.
			Day 5: Minor spotting. 1 mini pad all day.
Apr.17/96	22	4	*Day 1:* Minor dark spotting. 1 mini pad all day.
			Day 2: A bit more spotting.
			Day 3: Very light period.
			Day 4: Minimal bleeding.
			etc. **Start next line on the 1st day of your next period.**
May 15/96	28		*Day 1:*

Date of 1st day of menstrual period	# of days since 1st day of last period	# of days period duration	Nature of menstrual flow (amount, colour, density)

5
ASSESSING THE CURRENT STATE OF YOUR HEALTH

It is important at this stage in your life to take detailed stock of your health. Not just how you feel on the outside, but how healthy all your vital organs are on the inside. This will require your patience and perseverance in having numerous medical tests. It will also require a supportive medical partner.

STEP 2: *Find a Health Practitioner You Trust who:*

- Will work in partnership with you

- Takes your questions and test requests seriously

- Takes time to listen

- Takes time to think

- Is not drug-oriented

- Respects the value of alternative healthcare solutions and perhaps has training and knowledge in this area

- Is willing to provide you with copies of all your test results, and take the time to go through them with you in detail

- Is connected with good specialists, and will send you to them

This is a tall order. Take your time to find such a person, if you don't already have one.

STEP 3: *Complete the Process of Medical Testing.*

This is the first *big* step and it is critical to the future of your health. It may take some time to complete, but it could mean the difference between discovering and gently correcting a minor health problem now, and coping with a full-blown health crisis later.

WHY HAVE MEDICAL TESTS?

1. ***To make sure that your symptoms are those of menopause and not an illness***

    e.g. Fatigue, anxiety, restlessness, and sleeplessness can occur during menopause. They are also symptoms of hyperthyroidism, an overactive thyroid gland condition which can lead to congestive heart failure, if not properly treated.

    e.g. Fatigue and frequent urination can be symptoms of menopause. They are also symptoms of adult-onset diabetes.

2. ***To keep on top of menopausal symptoms which can lead to serious health problems if left untreated***

    e.g. Missed menstrual periods can sometimes lead to endometrial hyperplasia, a build-up of the lining of the uterus. When menstrual periods do start again, and the built-up blood is released, heavy bleeding can lead to iron-deficiency anemia.

    e.g. Surges in estrogen can lead to growth in uterine fibroids and ovarian cysts. These can cause pelvic pain, discomfort with sexual intercourse, pressure on the bladder, and heavy bleeding. Cysts can also turn cancerous. If cysts or fibroids grow too large, medical intervention may be required.

3. ***To identify your body's areas of potential future weakness, so that you can take action now to improve your long-term health prospects, without drugs***

    e.g. Blood pressure, cholesterol, triglyceride, and electrocardiogram tests can alert you to your risk of cardiovascular disease (heart and arteries).

    e.g. A bone density X-ray contributes one piece to the puzzle of predicting your risk of developing osteoporosis and experiencing bone fracture in the future.

RECOMMENDED MEDICAL TESTS

The Test Checklist at the end of this chapter lists recommended medical tests. For best results, follow the test process outlined in the box on the next page.

The most appropriate type of doctor or specialist to perform each test is indicated at the beginning of each test section. A suggested frequency of testing is indicated at the end of each test section.

The most accurate blood test results will be obtained if you do not eat or drink anything other than water for at least 12 hours prior to blood samples being taken.

More information about the tests relating to menopause, cardiovascular disease, and osteoporosis can be found in Chapter 6, "Understanding Your Test Results".

Test Process

1. Take the Test Checklist to your health practitioner and ask her or him to act as co-ordinator, to either perform the tests or refer you to the appropriate specialist(s). Your health practitioner will probably be your family doctor or another trained healthcare provider on whom you rely for general health care.

   Many of the tests are done in your doctor's office, as standard procedure during regular general check-ups. Others must be performed by specialists.

2. Before making an appointment for a test, read the relevant section under "Test Preparation Information" below. Helpful hints have been provided to ensure the most meaningful results.

3. Enter the test date in the appropriate space on the Test Checklist.

4. Obtain a copy of all test results. If necessary, borrow the originals from your family doctor or the specialist(s), and take them away to photocopy. In the case of the bone density X-ray, ask the technician to send an extra copy to your doctor, for you.

5. Enter the date when each test result was discussed with your doctor, and a brief note regarding any follow-up necessary.

TEST PREPARATION INFORMATION

Climacteric/Menopause ⇨ Family doctor to test

From the results of the four blood tests listed in the Test Checklist, you are looking for answers to the following two questions:

1. *Are you going through the climacteric (menopause)?*

   Remember, this is a time of hormonal change which can cause disruptive symptoms. If the answer is "Yes", it helps to explain your symptoms.

   The climacteric is diagnosed through body levels of estrogen and progesterone.

2. *Are you post-menopausal?*

   In other words, have you had your final menstrual period?

   This is determined through body levels of LH and FSH.

LH (luteinizing hormone) and FSH (follicle-stimulating hormone) are hormones which work together with estrogen to cause ovulation. When this teamwork breaks down because your egg supply has run out, you are post-menopausal.

The first question is the most difficult question to answer. The climacteric is often misdiagnosed.

Difficulties Diagnosing the Climacteric

Your doctor might order only LH and FSH tests, in response to your question as to whether or not you are going through the climacteric. However, knowledge of LH and FSH levels are only useful in determining whether a woman is post-menopausal, not whether she is going through the climacteric. By the time LH and FSH reach post-menopausal levels, most women will have been experiencing symptoms of the climacteric for a number of years.

If you are still having menstrual periods, and you are experiencing any of the symptoms described in Chapter 2, you will want to try to satisfy yourself that your symptoms are climacteric-related.

Technically, this requires a series of estrogen and progesterone hormone level tests, every two to three days over a menstrual cycle. But this would be expensive and inconvenient, since the standard method of checking hormone levels is through blood tests. It would mean a trip to the doctor's office, or the medical laboratory, every two to three days for about a month. Instead, most doctors try to diagnose the climacteric through a one-time set of blood tests.

But "one-shot" blood tests often give "false negative" results. That is, they may not confirm that you are going through the climacteric, when you really are.

It is not easy to diagnose the climacteric through "one-shot" blood test, for the following reasons:

- Timing of the blood tests often does not coincide with a time of noticeably out-of-sync hormone levels.

- Many women experience symptoms even with minor, unnoticeable hormone changes.

- Without the benefit of individual historical information, it is impossible to know whether a particular woman's current hormone levels reflect a variation from what has been "normal" for her.

Therefore, don't be too dismayed if your doctor declares, on the basis of a "one-shot" set of blood tests, that you are not going through menopause.

When to Book Your "One-Shot" Blood Tests for Better Chance of Accurate Results

Book your appointment for the "one-shot" estrogen, progesterone, LH and FSH blood tests so that it falls *14 days after the first day of your last menstrual period*. This is when your estrogen level would be at its peak, in a regular, non-climacteric menstrual cycle.

It is important to remember exactly where you were in your menstrual cycle on the day you had the blood tests, because "normal" levels for all hormones depend on where you are in your menstrual cycle. More about that in Chapter 6, "Understanding Your Test Results".

Test Frequency

To diagnose the climacteric: Preferably, have estrogen and progesterone levels tested every two to three days, at the same time each day, over one menstrual cycle. Otherwise, test estrogen, progesterone, LH, and FSH levels as agreed with your doctor.

To diagnose menopause: Have estrogen, progesterone, LH, and FSH levels tested when it has been at least 6 months since your last menstrual period.

Saliva Hormone Testing–Something New

A new, more convenient, and less invasive medical technique of hormone testing is now available in the United States and, on a very limited basis, in Canada. The method involves collecting saliva samples, in your own home, every few days, over one menstrual cycle.

I recently had my own hormone levels checked through the saliva testing technique, by collecting 11 saliva samples over 45 days (I don't have regular cycles anymore) and forwarding them through my doctor, for hormone testing.

The results were provided in data and graph form. Eleven points were plotted on the graph for each of estrogen and progesterone. The results confirmed what I had concluded from my menstrual period tracking records and my subsiding symptoms - I am very close to being post-menopausal.

The saliva testing technique is not yet available through a Canadian laboratory, nor is the approximate $250 cost covered by Canadian provincial health plans.

Cardiovascular (Heart & Arteries) ⇨ Family doctor to test

These tests will assess your risk of developing cardiovascular disease, which can lead to stroke and heart attack. For more accurate cholesterol readings, avoid consuming alcohol for 24 hours before the blood tests, and do not consume anything other than water for 12 hours before the blood tests.

Test Frequency

Annually, unless recommended more frequently by your doctor.

Bones ⇨ Technician at Bone Densitometry Centre to X-Ray

This test measures your bone density, usually at the hip and spine. Bone density is one of the factors currently considered to comprise part of your risk profile for developing osteoporosis and experiencing bone fracture. (Refer to Chapter 9, "Osteoporosis & Bone Fracture", for further discussion.)

The X-ray is taken by a specially trained technician. The level of radiation is extremely low. The test is simple, quick, non-invasive, and painless. You don't even have to undress.

Test Frequency

If the first X-ray shows that you have high bone density: Have the test every other year until your final menstrual period. After that, have the test annually for the next five years. After that, as advised by your doctor.

If the first X-ray shows that you have low bone density: Have the test annually, indefinitely, to monitor. Discuss with your doctor.

Ask the technician to send an extra copy of the test results to your doctor, for you.

Breasts

Mammograms are X-rays that check for breast abnormalities. In the newest mammogram equipment there is very low radiation and very little cancer risk.

In her book, *Dr. Susan Love's Breast Book*, Dr. Love says that mammograms before menopause are not as accurate in detecting breast cancer as those after menopause because, in most women, breast tissue is dense before menopause and fatty after menopause, and cancer shows up against fatty breast tissue but not against dense breast tissue.

Because of this tissue difference, mammograms have been successful in reducing mortality in post-menopausal women (due to early detection), but less so in pre-menopausal women (although some pre-menopausal women do have more fatty breast tissue and would derive early detection benefit from more frequent mammograms).

Breast tissue is also, generally, more dense during the last 14 days of the menstrual cycle. Therefore, for best results, mammograms should not be booked during those days.

It is preferable to have your mammogram done at a breast Screening Centre which:

- Specializes in mammography

- Has an radiological technologist (person who takes the pictures) who is specially trained in mammography and does nothing but mammograms

- Has a radiologist (doctor) who is specially trained to read mammograms and is considered an expert in the field

In Canada, The Canadian Association of Radiologists operates an accreditation program for mammography Screening Centres. Accreditation of a Screening Centre is based on quality of equipment, continuing medical education of technologists and radiologists, and review and assessment of patient diagnoses. Each Screening Centre is assessed for re-accreditation every three years.

The Canadian Association of Radiologists regularly publishes an updated list of accredited Screening Centres in Canada. The list can be found in both the Canadian Medical Journal and the Canadian Association of Radiologists Journal. You can obtain a copy of the list, or the location of an accredited Screening Centre convenient to you, by calling the Canadian Breast Cancer Foundation, toll free, at 1-800-387-9816.

In the United States, The American College of Radiology performs a similar accreditation function. For an accredited breast Screening Centre in your area call, toll free, 1-800-227-6440.

Before you go for your appointment, ask your doctor to advise the Screening Centre that you would like to have a verbal report, from the radiologist who reads your mammograms, immediately after the mammograms have been taken. In this way, you will not have to wait a week or so for the written report to get to your doctor and you will have an opportunity to ask questions of a specialist.

Test Frequency for Mammogram

From 40 years of age to menopause: Dr. Love recommends annual tests, if there is a strong family history of breast cancer. Otherwise, she considers every other year to be sufficient. The American Cancer Society recommends annual tests. The Canadian Cancer Society recommends that women 40-49 years of age discuss the need for mammogram with their doctor.

From menopause on: Dr. Love and The American Cancer Society recommend annual tests. The Canadian Cancer Society recommends that women age 50 and over have a mammogram every two years, or as recommended by their doctor.

A *Breast Physical Exam* should be performed once a year by each of your family doctor or trained healthcare provider and your gynecologist (to whom you go for physical examination of your reproductive organs). The purpose of this manual examination of your breasts is to check for irregularities and to cross-check the mammogram.

Breast Self-Examination (BSE) should also be performed by you, monthly, to learn what is normal for your breasts, and to monitor your breast health between mammograms and annual medical check-ups. Lumps can grow very quickly and become noticeable just months after a mammogram indicated nothing. The sooner breast cancer is discovered and treated, the higher the chance of full recovery.

It is important to know your breasts, so that you are aware of lumps or changes. And don't be shy about bringing these to the attention of your doctor. It is better to be safe than sorry.

Instructions for how to do BSE can be found at the end of this chapter, in a Canadian Breast Cancer Foundation publication entitled *The Easy Steps of Examining Your Own Breasts*.

Breast Health Reference

For excellent advice and facts on breast health care, read *Dr. Susan Love's Breast Book*, reference previously provided in Chapter 3.

Reproductive Organs ⇨ Gynecologist to test

A gynecologist specializes in the functions and diseases of the female reproductive system.

During a *Pelvic Exam* the gynecologist checks for abnormalities in the ovaries, fallopian tubes, uterus, cervix, and vagina. Fibroids, cysts, infection, and other abnormalities can be detected during a pelvic exam.

A *Pap Smear* is done during a pelvic exam. It is used to check the cervix (the lower part of the uterus) for pre-cancerous cells, cancerous cells, abnormal cell changes, infection, and sexually transmitted diseases. If caught and treated in the early stages, these problems almost never lead to anything serious.

An *Endometrial Biopsy* determines the health of the endometrium (the lining of the uterus), which can be adversely affected by hormonal imbalances. The gynecologist takes a small sample of the endometrial tissue to check for abnormal or cancerous cells.

During a *Transvaginal Ultrasound*, a technician places an ultrasound instrument inside the vagina. With this instrument, and its proximity to the reproductive organs, clearer pictures can better identify growths or abnormalities.

Test Frequency

Pelvic Exam:	Annually
Pap Smear:	Annually
Endometrial Biopsy:	Annually, if you are on estrogen but not progesterone replacement therapy. Otherwise once, and then on advice of gynecologist.
Transvaginal Ultrasound:	Annually

Colon ⇨ Gastroenterologist to test

A colonoscopy is a visual examination of the inside of the rectum and large intestine (colon) through a fibre-optic instrument with a lighted tip. It is performed by a gastroenterologist, a doctor specializing in the diagnosis and treatment of diseases of the gastrointestinal tract.

Changing hormone levels can cause intestinal upset and changes in bowel function. These symptoms can also signal problems such as an intestinal infection or the early stages of colon cancer. Intestinal infection, colitis, hemorrhoids, benign or cancerous tumours, and pre-cancerous polyps can all be discovered through a colonoscopy.

This test has a bad reputation for being painful. With a skilled specialist, it is painless, easy, and takes about 20 minutes (plus another couple of hours to recover from sedation). Find someone who has had a painless experience with this test, and ask your doctor make an appointment for you with the same gastroenterologist.

Test Frequency

Once, and then on advice of gastroenterologist, depending on results of colonoscopy.

Bladder/Kidneys/Adrenals/Liver ⇨ Family doctor to test

Changing hormone levels can temporarily affect the functioning of your bladder, kidneys, adrenal glands, and liver. Blood and urine tests should check for bladder or kidney infections and for the level of function of each organ.

Test Frequency

Annually, unless symptoms of infection arise in the interim.

Iron-Deficiency Anemia ⇨ Family doctor to test

Iron-deficiency anemia can result from the heavy and prolonged menstrual bleeding which often occurs during the climacteric. It reflects an inadequate supply of hemoglobin in the blood cells. Hemoglobin is the substance in the blood which carries oxygen from the lungs to body tissues. Without enough oxygen, you will feel tired, "low", and mentally slow.

The amount of ferritin in the blood is an indication of the body's underlying iron stores.

Low hemoglobin and ferritin levels leave the body tired, weak and vulnerable to infection and disease.

Test Frequency

Annually, unless heavy bleeding or fatigue indicate more frequent monitoring is necessary.

Diabetes ⇨ Family doctor to test

Adult-onset diabetes shares the symptoms of fatigue and frequent urination with the climacteric. Every woman should be tested for diabetes at this stage in her life.

Test Frequency

Once, and after that, depending on symptoms.

Hypothyroidism and Hyperthyroidism ⇨ Family doctor to test

Hypothyroidism is the condition of an underactive thyroid gland and Hyperthyroidism is the condition of an overactive thyroid gland. Both conditions share symptoms with the climacteric. Women with hypothyroidism can experience depression, mental impairment, poor memory, menstrual disorders, and many other symptoms. Women with Hyperthyroidism can experience fatigue, sleeplessness, sweating, accelerated bone loss, and many other symptoms. These conditions should both be tested for, as a matter of course.

Test Frequency

Annually

NOTES TO THE TEST CHECKLIST

1. This is not to be considered a comprehensive list to cover all possible health eventualities. The tests listed in the Test Checklist should be performed, at a minimum. Your doctor may suggest additional tests.

2. If you are experiencing unusual symptoms in areas not covered in this checklist (e.g., vision, hearing), make an appointment with a specialist in the respective field and have those symptoms assessed. Enter the test information at the bottom of the Test Checklist, on one of the blank rows.

TEST CHECKLIST

	Test	Test Type	Test Date	Date Results Discussed	Follow-up Required
Climacteric/ Menopause	Estrogen	Blood			
	Progesterone	Blood			
	LH	Blood			
	FSH	Blood			
Cardiovascular (Heart & Arteries)	Blood Pressure	External			
	Total Cholesterol	Blood			
	HDL Ratio	Blood			
	Triglycerides	Blood			
	Electrocardiogram (EKG)	Electrodes			
Bones	Bone Densitometry	X-ray			
Breasts	Mammogram	X-ray			
	Breast Physical Exam	Manual by Doctor			
	Breast Self-Examination	Manual by You			
Reproductive Organs	Pelvic Exam	Internal & External			
	Pap Smear	Internal			
	Endometrial Biopsy	Internal			
	Transvaginal Ultrasound	Internal			

TEST CHECKLIST (*Continued*)

Test	Test Type	Test Date	Date Results Discussed	Follow-up Required
Colon	Colonoscopy			
Bladder	Infection			
Kidneys	Infection/Protein/Function			
Adrenal Glands	Function			
Liver	Function			
Iron-Deficiency Anemia	Hemoglobin			
	Ferritin			
Diabetes	Glucose (Blood Sugar)			
Hypothyroidism	Thyroid function			
Hyperthyroidism	Thyroid function			

THE EASY STEPS OF EXAMINING YOUR OWN BREASTS

▷ IT ONLY TAKES A COUPLE OF MINUTES

&

▷ YOU ONLY DO IT ONCE A MONTH

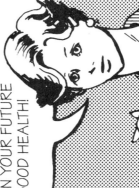

LET ME SHOW YOU HOW EASY IT IS!

MORE THINGS YOU SHOULD KNOW ABOUT
BREAST CANCER

▷ 1. EIGHTY PERCENT of breast lumps are not cancer. But only your doctor can tell. So if you find a lump or any change in your breasts, see your doctor right away.

▷ 2. Your doctor may suggest a Mammogram. Mammography can detect problems while they are still too small to be felt or seen – and help identify existing ones. *Modern Mammography machines give very low doses of radiation, so the procedure has very little risk.*

▷ 3. The only sure way to identify a breast lump is through a *biopsy* (microscope examination of a tissue sample).

▷ 4. If breast cancer is small and hasn't spread, the 10-year cure rate is about 90%! *Now you know how important it is to examine your breasts every month so problems can be caught early.*

▷ 5. Examine your breasts, both by sight and touch, *every month shortly after your period ends.* After menopause, do it at *the same time every month.* Have your breasts checked by your doctor at least once a year – preferably when you have your Pap Test. *And always check out any unusual findings right away!*

Courtesy of:
CANADIAN BREAST CANCER FOUNDATION
790 Bay St., Ste #1000, Toronto, Ontario M5G 1N8
Tel (416) 596-6773 or 1-800-387-9816
Special thanks to:
THE REGIONAL WOMEN'S HEALTH CENTRE
WOMEN'S COLLEGE HOSPITAL for providing translations, and
ST. MICHAEL'S HOSPITAL for technical advice.

Available in French, Cantonese, Greek, Italian, Portuguese, Polish, Farsi and Finnish
Concept and Writing: Patricia Harvie. Design and Drawings: Katherine Brown
Mechanical and Typesetting, Designers Inc.
Printing: Daughters of Penelope – Canadian Chapters

BEFORE YOU BEGIN

Remember, you are doing this examination so you will know what is normal for your breasts.

That way, you will quickly be able to spot any little changes – sores, lumps, indentations or nipple changes.

▷

READY NOW?

Open this folder to the inside and place it flat in front of you, so it is easy to see as you go.

Start at TOP LEFT and just follow the pictures.

▷

THINK OF THIS PROCEDURE AS "TAKING OUT LIFE INSURANCE" ON YOUR FUTURE GOOD HEALTH!

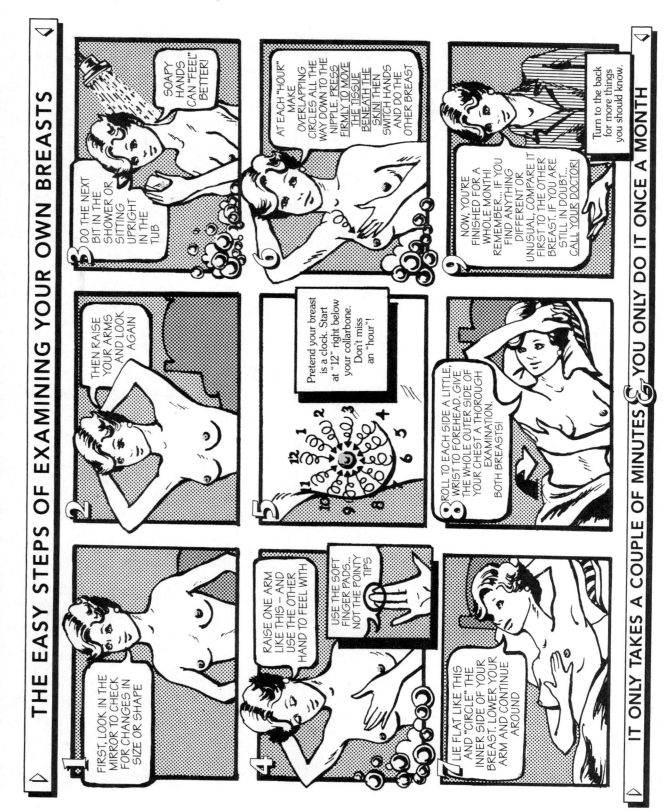

6
UNDERSTANDING YOUR TEST RESULTS

Understanding your test results will improve your chances of enjoying the best health care. Your test results should identify current and potential areas of weakness in your health, if any. To live a longer, healthier life you must be aware of those weaknesses and take action now to prevent serious health problems later.

STEP 4: *Identify Your Health Vulnerabilities.*

It is important to take unhurried time with your doctor to review your test results. Ask the secretary to have an extra copy of all test results available for you, prior to the appointment.

Discuss each individual test result with your doctor. Ask for explanations. Keep your copy of the results in a file. The next time you have the tests, you will be able to compare and watch for negative trends. For many health problems, catching them in the early stages allows time for curing or alleviating them through gentler means than drugs or surgery.

This chapter focuses on interpreting the results of tests specific to the process of the climacteric, and to the major health risks associated with lower post-menopausal hormone levels - cardiovascular disease and osteoporosis. It may become a bit technical at times. Reread it, if necessary. It is worth understanding.

Specific test results will be discussed for:

☞ **Climacteric/Menopause**

☞ **Cardiovascular**

☞ **Bones**

☞ CLIMACTERIC/MENOPAUSE

As indicated in Chapter 5, from the results of the four blood tests, you are looking for answers to the following two questions:

1. *Are you going through the climacteric (menopause)?*

2. *Are you post-menopausal?*

Estrogen & Progesterone are the Key to the Climacteric

Estrogen and progesterone levels are the most important indicators of whether a woman is going through menopause. These hormone levels go through periods of wide swings, imbalance, and reduction for years before a woman's final menstrual period.

As also indicated in Chapter 5, it is difficult to accurately diagnose whether a woman's symptoms are caused by menopause-related hormone changes, based on the results of "one-shot" blood tests. A series of estrogen and progesterone hormone tests is usually required.

LH and FSH are the Key to Post-Menopause

LH and FSH levels, taken together, are indicators of whether a woman is close to, or past, her final menstrual period (i.e., post-menopausal). They are not indicators of whether a woman is going through menopause.

Understanding Hormone Blood Test Results Data

The format and standard measures of hormone blood test results vary depending on the laboratory to which the blood samples are sent for analysis. They also differ by country.

An example of what hormone blood test results can look like is provided in the box on the next page. The Blood Levels provided are my blood levels, at a difficult point in time during my menopausal years. The blood tests were taken 14 days after the first day of a menstrual period.

Hormone	My 1994 Blood Level	Time in Cycle	Normal Range
Estradiol (Estrogen)	**410**	Follicular **Mid-Cycle** Luteal Post-Menopausal Pre-Pubertal Children	110 - 550 pmol/l 550 - 1650 pmol/l 180 - 845 pmol/l less than 100 pmol/l 37 - 92 pmol/l
		(Note that post-menopausal estrogen levels are similar to pre-pubertal estrogen levels.)	
Progesterone	**15.8**	Follicular Luteal Post-Menopausal	0.6 - 2.6 nmol/l 13.2 - 75.2 nmol/l 0.4 - 1.8 nmol/l
LH	**4**	Follicular Mid-Cycle Luteal Post-Menopausal	1 - 26 iu/l 25 - 57 iu/l 1 - 27 iu/l 40 - 104 iu/l
FSH	**12**	Follicular Mid-Cycle Luteal Post-Menopausal	1 - 10 iu/l 2 - 21 iu/l 1 - 8 iu/l 34 - 96 iu/l

What is considered to be a "normal" blood level, for a particular hormone, depends on when in the menstrual cycle the blood test was taken ("Time in Cycle"). The Sample Hormone Tracking Chart on the next page shows the approximate division of the menstrual cycle into three phases: Follicular, Mid-Cycle, Luteal.

The Sample Hormone Tracking Chart also roughly illustrates the typical rise and fall of estrogen and progesterone over a normal, pre-climacteric, pre-menopausal, menstrual cycle. As you can see, estrogen and progesterone levels also change within each phase in the cycle. As well, "normal" levels vary from woman to woman.

Using my own 1994 hormone levels shown in the box above as an example, the estrogen (410) and progesterone (15.8) levels have been plotted, at the 14 Day mark, on the Sample Hormone Tracking Chart on the next page. (The explanation at the bottom of the chart describes how.)

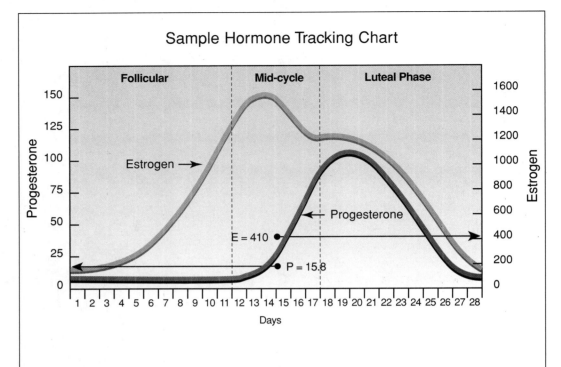

Sample Hormone Tracking Chart

Explanation:

1. The estrogen level of 410 has been plotted above the 14 Day mark,
    using the Estrogen scale on the right side of the chart to determine how
    high up to plot the number.

2. The progesterone level of 15.8 has been plotted above the 14 Day mark,
    using the Progesterone scale on the left side of the chart to determine
    how high up to plot the number.

For that time in the cycle, my *progesterone* level was "normal"; but my *estrogen* level
was very low. Estrogen at mid-cycle would "normally" be much higher, up in the
vicinity of where the graph line peaks, closer to the top of the chart. These test results,
coupled with my symptoms, confirmed hormonal imbalance as the cause of my
suffering- at least, they did to me at the time.

By way of comparison, and subsequent to the above blood tests, I had my hormone
levels tested about a week after I started taking Dong Quai (a Chinese menopause herb
referred to in Chapter 7). Those blood samples were taken on Day 17 of a menstrual
cycle, and showed my estrogen level at 1550.

Note also that my blood levels of LH and FSH indicated that I was not post-
menopausal.

See the next section for instructions for setting up and plotting your own hormone
tracking chart.

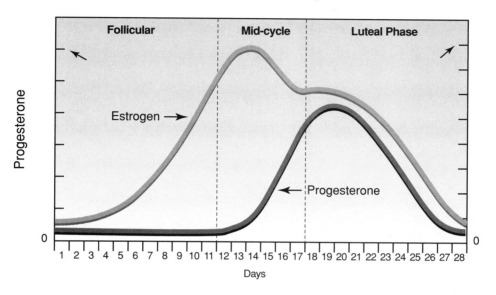

Your Hormone Tracking Chart

Instructions:

1. Set up the right axis scale (the Estrogen axis) by placing the highest number, from the Estrogen (Estradiol) "normal range" on your test results sheet, at the highest axis marker as shown by the arrow at the upper right side of the chart.

2. Number each of the Estrogen axis markers in equivalent steps down to the zero at the bottom.

3. Set up the left axis scale (the Progesterone axis) by placing the highest number, from the Progesterone "normal range" on your test results sheet, at the highest axis marker as shown by the arrow at the upper left side of the chart.

4. Number each of the Progesterone axis markers in equivalent steps down to the zero at the bottom.

5. Go to the Day number (along the bottom) which represents the number of days after the start of your last menstrual period that you had the hormone tests.

6. Plot your Estrogen level above that Day and up the right side scale at the level indicated on your test results.

7. Plot your Progesterone level above that Day and up the left side scale at the level indicated on your test results.

Setting Up and Plotting Your Own Hormone Tracking Chart

Regardless of the standard of measurement used by your laboratory, the idea is generally the same. Now you can set-up and plot your own estrogen and progesterone levels on Your Hormone Tracking Chart on the previous page. Follow the instructions at the bottom of the chart.

Each time you have estrogen and progesterone levels measured, plot the results on Your Hormone Tracking Chart. You will probably see inconsistent levels over time. That is indicative of a time of hormonal change. As you come closer to your final menstrual period, your estrogen and progesterone levels will decline to very low levels and remain there.

Remember, test results which show close to "normal" hormone levels do not necessarily mean that you are not going through the climacteric, or that your symptoms are not caused by hormonal imbalances or changes. Such results may mean that your hormones have not been measured at a time when they were noticeably out of balance, or out of the "normal" range.

If your menstrual periods are changing (review what you have recorded in your tracking records), and you are experiencing other symptoms, such as any of those outlined in Chapter 2, you are most likely going through menopause, or experiencing hormonal changes or imbalances.

☞ CARDIOVASCULAR

The cardiovascular tests outlined in the Test Checklist in Chapter 5 will give your doctor enough information to determine whether your cardiovascular system (heart and arteries) is healthy. If these tests show that it is healthy, no further tests will be required. If not, further tests may be required, and diet and lifestyle changes (outlined in Chapter 8, "Improving Your Long-Term Health Prospects") will be necessary to ensure a longer, healthier life.

Explanations of how to interpret the results of the tests are provided below, based primarily on information from the following book by U.S. heart specialist, Dr. John McDougall. Dr. McDougall's book also outlines those further tests which may be necessary, if cardiovascular problems are detected.

Title:	*The McDougall Program for a Healthy Heart*
Author:	John A. McDougall, M.D.
Published:	1996
Publisher:	Penguin Books
ISBN:	0-525-93868-0
Reference:	Chapter 11, pages 142-170

Blood Pressure

High blood pressure (also called hypertension) is an indicator of trouble in blood circulation. High blood pressure can lead to stroke, heart attack, congestive heart failure, and kidney disease.

Blood pressure is the force required to pump oxygen and nutrient-laden blood to different parts of the body. The more flexible (healthy) your arteries, the lower your blood pressure. The harder (more unhealthy) your arteries, the higher your blood pressure and the greater your risk of stroke, heart attack, and other health problems.

Ask your doctor what your blood pressure is. The box below provides an interpretation for each reading. (For 110/70 - read : one hundred and ten over seventy.)

Resting Blood Pressure (without medication)	Interpretation
110/70 or less :	Ideal.
120/80:	Considered the "normal" resting blood pressure.
140/90:	If the top number is greater than 140 or the bottom number is greater than 90, it is considered high blood pressure or hypertension.

Total Cholesterol

Your Total Cholesterol is made up primarily of HDL (high-density lipoprotein) cholesterol and LDL (low-density lipoprotein) cholesterol. LDLs contribute to the development of cardiovascular disease and HDLs help remove LDLs from the body. Therefore, the higher your HDLs, the lower your risk of cardiovascular disease.

There has been discussion in medical circles as to the importance of Total Cholesterol, alone, in determining cardiovascular health. The latest thinking is that Total Cholesterol should be viewed together with the HDL Ratio. If your Total Cholesterol is high but your HDL Ratio is low, it means there are lots of "good" HDLs available in your blood to remove the "bad" LDLs from your arteries. In this case, your risk of cardiovascular disease would be considered to be low (see HDL Ratio below).

It is still important to know your Total Cholesterol level. It does form part of the picture of your cardiovascular health and of the assessment of your risk of developing cardiovascular disease (which leads to heart attack or stroke). It is also considered a factor in your risk of contracting other diseases such as diabetes, cancer, and liver disease.

Also, be aware that when "Western" doctors talk about "normal" cholesterol levels, they are talking about what is *common* in the North American population. What is "normal" in North America, where the population generally consumes a high-fat, animal-based diet, is not "normal", for example, in China, where the population generally consumes a low-fat, plant-based diet (and has a much lower incidence of cardiovascular disease than in North America).[1] What is "normal" in North America for cholesterol, may not be healthy for you.

The box below provides an interpretation of each level of Total Cholesterol, primarily using Dr. McDougall's approach. (Equivalent Canadian values are provided in brackets.)

Total Cholesterol	Interpretation
less than 150 mg/dl (3.9 mmol/l):	Ideal. Little or no risk of heart attack or stroke. Chinese in China average 127 (3.30).[2]
151-179 mg/dl (3.91-4.63 mmol/l):	Low risk. A few diet and lifestyle changes would move you down into the safer range.
180-199 mg/dl (4.64-5.14 mmol/l):	Twice the heart attack risk of less than 180 mg/dl.
200-219 mg/dl (5.15-5.66 mmol/l):	Higher risk of heart attack and stroke. The U.S. national average is approximately 205 (5.33).[3]
220-239 mg/dl (5.67-6.18 mmol/l):	High. Requires immediate treatment.
240-299 mg/dl (6.19-7.73 mmol/l):	4 times the rate of heart attack and stroke of those at less than 200 mg/dl.
more than 300 mg/dl (7.74 mmol/l):	High risk of early death from heart attack or stroke.

HDL Ratio

Calculate your HDL Ratio by dividing your Total Cholesterol by your HDL cholesterol level. For example, if your Total Cholesterol is 200 mg/dl (5.15 mmol/l) and your HDL is 50 mg/dl (1.3 mmol/l), then your HDL Ratio is:

$$200 \div 50 = 4 \quad (5.15 \div 1.3 = 4).$$

Dr. William Castelli, medical director of the Framingham, Massachusetts Cardiovascular Institute considers the HDL Ratio to be a better predictor of risk of cardiovascular disease than Total Cholesterol.[4]

Find out what your HDL Ratio is and interpret it according to the definitions provided in the box below.

HDL Ratio	Interpretation
less than 3.0	Ideal.
3.0 - 4.0	Considered healthy.
greater than 4.0	As your HDL ratio increases above 4.0, your risk of heart attack and stroke increases.

Triglycerides

Triglycerides are fat circulating in the blood. Triglycerides can cause blood clots to form, thereby increasing the chance of heart attack or thrombosis (blood clot in vein or artery).

Healthy blood levels of triglycerides are as follows, according to Dr. McDougall:

Men	40 - 150mg/dl	(1.03 - 3.88 mmol/l)
Women	35 - 135mg/dl	(0.9 - 3.49 mmol/l)

Electrocardiogram (EKG/ECG)

This test checks the heart for a wide range of possible abnormalities, such as, rhythm, injury from heart attack, inflammation, and atherosclerosis.

☞ BONES

Bone Densitometry Test Results

In my opinion, the value of having bone density tests in the years surrounding your final menstrual period is fivefold:

- To determine your current bone mineral density (BMD), with which there is a high correlation to bone strength[5]

- To monitor your bone loss, if any, over time

- To project your bone density into the future, if your bone loss after menopause were to follow the perceived "common" pattern

- To contribute one piece to the puzzle of predicting your risk of developing osteoporosis and experiencing bone fracture in the future (Refer to Chapter 9, "Osteoporosis & Bone Fracture" for details.)

- To raise awareness, so you can start now to protect your bone health

According to a group of international researchers, bone densitometry is currently "the best approach to screen individuals for their risk of developing osteoporosis." [6]

Bone densitometry in Canada and in the United States is most often performed using one of the following two densitometry systems:

HOLOGIC   or   LUNAR

The rest of this section will explain bone densitometry reports. Refer to your own bone densitometry reports as you read through it.

Getting the Message from Your Bone Densitometry Reports

The Hologic and Lunar reports both provide the same basic information, but they are laid out differently. There is one report for your hip and one report for your spine. Each report has 3 components:

COMPONENT 1:   A picture of your spine or hip

COMPONENT 2:   A lot of data

COMPONENT 3:   A graph

COMPONENT 1: *The Picture*

The picture of your spine is divided into four regions: L1, L2, L3, L4. The X-ray is actually of your lumbar spine - the lower part of your spine. The procedure cannot accurately measure the upper part of the spine, where the compression occurs that causes "dowager's hump". The lower part of the spine is used as representative of what is happening in the upper part.

The picture of your hip has three main regions: Neck, Ward's (Triangle), Troch(anter). The Neck is identified in the picture by the long, narrow rectangle, super-imposed on top of it. The Ward's Triangle is identified by the small square, super-imposed within the Neck rectangle. The Trochanter is the section just below the Neck, including the rounded, bulbous part which protrudes out to the left or right, depending on which hip was X-rayed. Over 90% of hip fractures occur in either the Neck or the rounded, bulbous part.[7]

COMPONENT 2: *The Data*

Data is provided which allows you to:

- Know your current bone mineral density (BMD)

- Compare your current BMD to the BMD of a sample population of normal, healthy, pre-menopausal women

- Compare your current BMD to the BMD of a sample population of women, with non-chronic diseases or medications affecting bones; of your age, weight, and ethnic background; without fractures (African-Americans tend to have higher bone mass values and Asian ethnic groups tend to have lower bone mass values than Caucasians.)[8-12]

In the Hologic report, this data is found in a box that looks something like this, using a sample hip report as an example.

Region	BMD	T		Z	
Neck	0.745	-1.49	83%	-1.33	85%
Troch	0.612	-1.22	85%	-1.20	85%
Inter	1.032	-0.82	90%	-0.80	90%
TOTAL	0.866	-0.91	89%	-0.87	89%
Ward's	0.662	-1.21	83%	-0.71	89%

In the Lunar report, this data is found in a table that looks something like this, using *my* own hip report as an example:

Region	BMD g/cm²	Young Adult %	Young Adult Z	Age Matched %	Age Matched Z
Neck	0.830	85	-1.25	94	-0.47
Wards	0.770	85	-1.08	98	-0.10
Troch	0.707	90	-0.75	97	-0.23

Data Explanations

Definitions of the relevant data-related terms found in the reports are provided below. Terms outside the brackets are Hologic terms and inside the brackets (if they differ) are the equivalent Lunar terms. Refer to your own hip and spine densitometry reports.

- *BMD* is your actual bone mineral density for each region of your hip or spine. It is measured in grams per centimetre squared (g/cm²).

- *T* - % column (*Young Adult %*) values indicate what % your bone density is of the average bone density of a sample of normal, healthy, pre-menopausal women.

- *T* - column of numbers to left of the % column (*Young Adult Z*) values indicate the number of standard deviations your bone density is above or below the average bone density of the same sample of normal, healthy, pre-menopausal women. This is how much your bone density is greater than or less than the average for the sample of women to which you are being compared. (One standard deviation equals .10 g/cm² for Hologic and .12 g/cm² for Lunar.)

- *Z* - % column (*Age Matched %*) values indicate what % your bone density is of the average bone density of a sample of women, with non-chronic diseases or medications affecting bones; of your age, weight, and ethnic background; without fractures.

- *Z* - column of numbers to left of the % column (*Age Matched Z*) values indicate the number of standard deviations your bone density is above or below the average bone density of the same sample of women, with non-chronic diseases or medications affecting bones; of your age, weight, and ethnic background; without fractures. This is how much your bone density is greater than or less than the average for the sample of women to which you are being compared.

The only data that is relevant to your risk of developing osteoporosis and experiencing bone fracture is your own BMD. Comparisons to other sample populations may put your bone status into perspective, but they do not impact on your personal bone health. If the sample population to which you are being compared, in your post-menopausal age range, has low bone density, you can derive no comfort from being within the norm for that group.

COMPONENT 3: *The Graph*

The following graph illustrates the concept of what you will see on your own graphs. It does not look exactly like either the Hologic or the Lunar graphs, but contains features from each. Your graphs may be in colour, or black and white, depending on the printer at the Centre where you were tested. The asterisk plotted on the following graph represents the bone density of the Neck region of my left hip. The following explanation will help you interpret your graphs.

Graph Explanation

- The *asterisk* in the graph, corresponds to the *asterisk inside the white circle* on the graph in the Lunar report and to the "+" symbol on the graph in the Hologic report. This asterisk or "+", on your graphs, plots the actual bone mineral density of the *Neck* region of your hip, and the bone mineral density of your spine (BMD axis to the left), as at your age (AGE axis below).

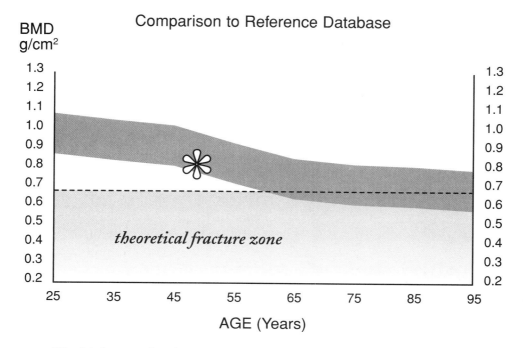

The higher up the chart your asterisk or "+", the more dense your bones. The lower down the chart your asterisk or "+", the more porous your bones.

As noted, the asterisk in the above graph above represents the bone density of the Neck region of my left hip. If you look back to page 59, to the Lunar report data table which provides my hip bone densities, you will see that my left hip Neck bone density was 0.830 g/cm² at the time of the test. I was 47 years old. Those are the two co-ordinates used to plot my asterisk on the above graph.

• The *thick band* running across and down to the right in the graph (inside which my asterisk happens to be located) corresponds to the *thick black band* (or blue, if it is in colour) on the graph in the Lunar report, and to the *thick double band* (or double blue, if it is in colour) on the graph in the Hologic report.

In approximately the 20-45 year age range, the band represents a range of BMD values for a small cross-sectional sample of normal, healthy, pre-menopausal women of your ethnic background. In approximately the 45+ year age range, the band represents a range of values for a small cross-sectional sample of women, with non-chronic diseases or medications affecting bones; of your age, weight, and ethnic background; without fractures.

The downward direction of the band reflects what was found to happen to bone density in 68% of the small cross-sectional sample population used to establish the comparison standards. It also reflects what has generally been found in research (see "Predicting Your Future Bone Density and Fracture Risk", later in this chapter).[13]

- The *line* drawn across the graph, below the 0.7 g/cm² mark, corresponds to the *midpoint of the bar* (yellow, if it is in colour) which runs just below the 0.74g/cm² line on the graph in the Lunar report and corresponds to the *broken line across the graph* in the Hologic report. This is the line below which you are considered to be osteoporotic.[14] The area below this line is called the "theoretical fracture zone". The further below the line your asterisk or "+" symbol, the higher your risk of fracture is considered to be.[15-17]

YOUR GOAL

KEEP YOUR BONE DENSITY AS FAR ABOVE THE LINE AS POSSIBLE

Predicting Your Future Bone Density and Fracture Risk

If we assume that we are all going to follow what has generally been accepted as the common pattern of post-menopausal bone loss (and as will later be discussed, this is not necessarily a valid assumption), we can predict the age at which our bone density will fall into the "theoretical fracture zone".

To do this, project your asterisk or "+" down and to the right on its graph, on the same angle as the thick band. At the point where your asterisk or "+" moves into the "theoretical fracture zone", look down to the AGE axis below to see how old you will be. This is the age at which you may be diagnosed as having osteoporosis, and at which your bones are expected to be at risk for easy fracture. My own hip should be osteoporotic at about age 57.

It May Not Happen to You

Predicting future bone density and fracture risk is not a perfect science. Three points should be noted.

1. The studies used to determine a "common" pattern for expected aging bone loss were almost all *cross-sectional studies*, in which bone densities were taken, at one point in time, of a *small sample* of women, of different ages and menopausal status. These bone densities were then allocated to groups based on the age and menopausal status of the women. Average bone densities were calculated for each group.

    A pattern emerged from these studies which showed generally lower bone densities in older women, with more rapidly reducing bone densities in women who were in the five or so years after menopause.[18] The validity of attributing this pattern to the entire female population is questionable, particularly in view of **2.** below.

Longitudinal studies are what we really need, but none has been completed of sufficient size or duration to draw valid conclusions about patterns for longer-term bone density changes and actual fracture occurrence. Longitudinal studies would take a sample of women, of different ages and menopausal status, and track their individual bone densities, over time, to determine each woman's pattern of bone density, with aging and changing menopausal status. The results would then be used to draw conclusions about the general population. We need to study what happens to the bones of a very large sample of women, with different habits, diets, lifestyles, and ethnic backgrounds, over a long period of time, as they go from say 30 to 90 years old. This would be a better approach to determining a common pattern, if there is one.

2. Even if there is a "common" pattern of bone loss after menopause, many women do not fit into it. In fact, some women *add*! bone density in the years after menopause.[19,20]

3. Some women, whose bone density has declined well into the "theoretical fracture zone", do not experience bone fracture, even after falling.[21]

So Don't Panic!

There is no urgency for most women to take hormone replacement therapy (HRT) to reduce their risk of developing osteoporosis, and possibly experiencing bone fracture some 10-30 years in the future. There are many factors involved in the development of osteoporosis and in the actual occurrence of bone fracture. Reduced female hormone production is only one possible factor.

Research continues to fill in the gaps in our knowledge of what causes bone fracture in elderly people. Perhaps someday soon there will be less destructive ways than serious drugs to protect our bone health as we age. To be sure, taking HRT does *not guarantee* protection from osteoporosis or bone fracture.

In the meantime, we can each take action to protect our own bone health through diet, exercise, and lifestyle. Chapter 8, "Improving Your Long-Term Health Prospects" and Chapter 9, "Osteoporosis & Bone Fracture" will help you develop a plan of action.

References

1. Chen, J., Campbell, T. C., Li J., Peto, R. *Diet, Life-style and Mortality in China: A Study of the Characteristics of 65 Chinese Counties.* Oxford: Oxford University Press, 1990, pp. 49-52.
2. Ibid.
3. National Health and Nutrition Examination Surveys (NHANES III, conducted in 1990). Cited in Ernst, N. D., Sempos, C. T., Briefel, R. R., and Clark, M. "Consistency between US dietary fat intake and serum total cholesterol concentrations: the National Health and Nutrition Examination Surveys." *American Journal of Clinical Nutrition* 1997; 66(suppl): 965S-972S.
4. As advised in an article entitled "Do Your Heart Good" by Cathy Perlmutter with Susan C. Smith, Ed Slaughter, and Toby Hanlon in *Prevention* magazine, February, 1997, p. 82.
5. Johnston, C. C. Jr. and Melton, L. J. III. "Bone Densitometry." In *Osteoporosis: Etiology, Diagnosis, and Management*, Riggs, B. L. and Melton, L. J. III (eds.). 2nd Edition, Philadelphia:Lippincott-Raven, 1995, pp. 275-297.
6. Peck, W.A., Burckhardt, P., Christiansen, C., et al. "Consensus development conference: diagnosis, prophylaxis, and treatment of osteoporosis." *American Journal of Medicine* 1993; 94:646-650.
7. Zuckerman, J. D. "Hip Fracture." *The New England Journal of Medicine* 1996; 334 (23): 1519-1525.
8. Tobias, J. H., Cook, D. G., Chambers, T. J., and Dalzell, N. "A comparison of bone mineral density between Caucasian, Asian and Afro-Caribbean women." *Clinical Science* 1994; 87:587-591.
9. DeSimone, D. P., Stevens, J., Edwards, J., Shary, J., Gordon, L., and Bell, N. H. "Influence of Body Habitus and Race on Bone Mineral Density of the Midradius, Hip, and Spine in Aging Women." *Journal of Bone and Mineral Research* 1989; 4 (6): 827-830.
10. Liel, Y., Edwards, J., Shary, J., Spicer, K. M., Gordon, L., and Bell, N. H. "The Effects of Race and Body Habitus on Bone Mineral Density of the Radius, Hip, and Spine in Premenopausal Women." *Journal of Clinical Endocrinology and Metabolism* 1988; 66 (6): 1247-1250.
11. Luckey, M. M., Meier, D. E., Mandeli, J. P., DaCosta, M. C., Hubbard, M. L., and Goldsmith, S. J. "Radial and Vertebral Bone Density in White and Black Women: Evidence for Racial Differences in Premenopausal Bone Homeostasis." *Journal of Clinical Endocrinology and Metabolism* 1989; 69 (4): 762-770.
12. Kleerekoper, M., Nelson, D. A., Peterson, E. L., Flynn, M. J., Pawluszka. A. S., Jacobsen, G., and Wilson, P. "Reference Data for Bone Mass, Calciotropic Hormones, and Biochemical Markers of Bone Remodeling in Older (55-75) Postmenopausal White and Black Women." *Journal of Bone and Mineral Research* 1994; 9 (8): 1267-1276.
13. Lindsay, R. "Estrogen Deficiency." In *Osteoporosis: Etiology, Diagnosis, and Management*, Riggs, B. L. and Melton, L. J. III (eds.). 2nd Edition, Philadelphia: Lippincott-Raven, 1995, pp. 133-160.

14. Kanis, J. A., Melton, L. J. III, Christiansen, C., Johnston, C. C. and Khaltaev, N. "Perspective : The Diagnosis of Osteoporosis." *Journal of Bone and Mineral Research* 1994; 9 (8): 1137-1141.

15. Riggs, B. L. and Melton, L. J. III. "Medical progress: involutional osteoporosis." *New England Journal of Medicine* 1986; 314:1676-1686.

16. Greenspan, S. L., Myers, E. R., Maitland, L. A., Resnick, N. M., and Hayes, W. C. "Fall severity and bone mineral density as risk factors for hip fracture in ambulatory elderly." *Journal of American Medical Association* 1994; 271:128-133.

17. Cummings, S. R., Black, D. M., Nevitt, M. C., Browner, W., Cauley, J., Ensrud, K., Genant, H. K., Palermo, L., Scott, J., and Vogt, T. M. for the Study of Osteoporotic Fractures Research Group. "Bone density at various sites for prediction of hip fractures." *Lancet* 1993; 341:72-75.

18. Lindsay, R. "Estrogen Deficiency." In *Osteoporosis: Etiology, Diagnosis, and Management*, Riggs, B. L. and Melton, L. J. III (eds.). 2nd Edition, Philadelphia: Lippincott-Raven, 1995, pp. 133-160.

19. Harris, S. and Dawson-Hughes, B. "Rates of change in bone mineral density of spine, heel, femoral neck and radius in healthy postmenopausal women." *Bone and Mineral* 1992; 17: 87-95.

20. Pouilles, J. M., Tremollieres, F. and Ribot, C. "The Effects of Menopause on Longitudinal Bone Loss from the Spine." *Calcified Tissue International* 1993; 52: 340-343.

21. Greenspan, S. L., Myers, E. R., Maitland, L. A., Resnick, N. M., and Hayes, W. C. "Fall severity and bone mineral density as risk factors for hip fracture in ambulatory elderly." *Journal of American Medical Association* 1994; 271:128-133.

7

GETTING THROUGH THE MENOPAUSAL YEARS WITHOUT DRUGS

Getting through the menopausal years without drugs is by far the greatest challenge for women who must maintain a high level of performance during the most demanding time in their lives. Income-earning responsibilities, child-rearing concerns, and ailing elderly relatives combine to make the mid-life years for women a time of peak demand on their physical, emotional, and intellectual capacities.

For many women, menopausal symptoms cause a decrease in capacity and productivity at a time when they can least afford it. Although most symptoms are temporary, they are not necessarily brief, and the exact duration cannot be known in advance. This is not two to three days a month of PMS or nine months of pregnancy. The most disruptive symptoms seem to last about two to three years, but everyone is different and there is no specific timeframe. You cannot count the days or make plans.

Many women risk their long-term health by taking hormone replacement therapy (HRT) as an immediate solution to an immediate problem. This is primarily because they turn for help to their doctors, who are usually unaware of non-drug alternatives. Unfortunately, the side effects of HRT cause many women to stop taking the drugs within the first year. Symptoms then return, often at a more severe level.

This chapter will help you find non-drug ways to reduce the severity of your menopausal symptoms. Non-drug options for alleviating some of the most common difficult symptoms will be provided. Try non-drug methods first. They may be all you need to make it gently and safely through your menopausal years.

STEP 5: *Relieve Menopausal Symptoms without Drugs.*

Try alternative therapies such as:

☞   **Herbs**

☞   **Traditional Chinese Medicine**

☞   **Diet**

☞   **Exercise**

☞   HERBS

Plant herbs have provided effective treatment for human ailments for thousands of years. Of course, many of the chemical drugs of today have their origins in plant substances.

More and more, we are realizing the superiority of natural treatments over chemical drugs for many human afflictions. But treatments found in nature take longer to have an impact and can be harmful, if not used knowledgeably and with care. It is important to take herbs only under the direction of a trained naturopath or herbalist. Negative interactions can occur with other herbs and with drugs.

Naturopathy is a drugless system of treating the underlying cause of symptoms through natural means such as nutrition, herbs, sunlight, exercise, etc. It is a preventative approach to health care.

Many pharmacists today are certified naturopaths. You may find a pharmacist/naturopath in one of your own neighbourhood pharmacies. This would be a good resource individual for natural health care advice.

As a guide to herbal and other treatments for symptoms of the climacteric, the following book is recommended:

Title: *Menopausal Years: The Wise Woman Way*
Author: Susun S. Weed
Published: 1992
Publisher: Ash Tree Publishing
ISBN: 0-9614620-4-3

Menopausal Years: The Wise Woman Way is a comprehensive review of a wide range of remedies (herbal, chemical drug, surgery, and other) available for difficulties of the climacteric. The book contains many treatment options for each symptom; although, as a medicinal herbalist, Susun Weed's philosophy is strongly naturopathic.

For example, Susun recommends Stinging Nettle as a good all round herbal remedy for symptoms of the climacteric. Stinging Nettle is considered effective in reducing the severity of menopausal symptoms such as:

- Anxiety
- Fatigue
- Water retention
- Joint soreness
- Sleep disturbances
- Urinary tract problems

Stinging Nettle can be purchased in a health food store and, like most herbal remedies, can be taken in the form of an infusion or a tincture.

An herbal infusion is similar to an herbal tea, with a couple of differences. An infusion uses a much larger amount of a dried herb than a tea, and an infusion is brewed for much longer than a tea. This makes an herbal infusion stronger and more potent than an herbal tea.

An herbal tincture is a liquid which has been made by soaking fresh herbs in alcohol for at least 6 weeks. The liquid is then consumed in small amounts at a time by adding a prescribed number of drops to a small amount of water, and drinking.

Cautionary Notes About Herbs

- Herbs should be taken in moderation and under the care of a trained specialist.
- Start with lower doses and increase if necessary.
- If side-effects are experienced from taking a particular herb, stop taking it.
- *Do not take any herb for longer than a few months without a break.*

☞ TRADITIONAL CHINESE MEDICINE

Traditional Chinese Medicine (TCM) is an ancient form of healing which has been practised for over 5,000 years. It is the world's oldest and most comprehensive system of medical care. It is based on a philosophy that encompasses the well-being of the body and the soul.

The primary purpose of Chinese herbal medicine is to prevent disease. This is accomplished through the healthy diet and lifestyle of the patient, and the ability of the doctor to detect and treat diseases to which the patient is vulnerable, before they strike. (This is clearly the way North American health care should be heading, and it is the purpose behind the medical test recommendations outlined in Chapter 5, and the diet and lifestyle recommendations outlined in Chapter 8.)

Once disease strikes, TCM attempts to recognize and treat the underlying cause. It tries to identify what conditions have lowered the body's resistance and allowed disease to invade. When those conditions are corrected, disease is expected to disappear because it can no longer thrive. Treatment is initially through diet (including herbs) and lifestyle. If this fails, drugs are the next level of recourse.

A traditional Chinese doctor diagnoses a patient's underlying condition by reading his or her physical indicators through the four techniques of interviewing, observing, listening, and feeling.

If you go to a traditional Chinese doctor, she or he will interview you to gain knowledge of your personal health history and current symptoms. She will observe your complexion, eyes, tongue colour and texture, and other physical conditions. She will listen to your speech, breathing, coughing, and bodily sounds. She will feel your pulses and internal organs through finger pressure.

Chinese Herbs

If you plan to use Chinese herbs to try to reduce menopausal distress, you should do so under the care of a traditional Chinese doctor. Obtain a referral from someone whose judgement you trust, and for whom TCM has been successful.

Regular visits are necessary so that your condition can be monitored, and herbal treatments can be adjusted to meet the changing needs of your hormonal state.

Many of the Chinese herbs used to alleviate symptoms of menopause contain phytosterols. These are estrogen and progesterone hormones from plant (phyto) sources. These hormones are much milder than chemical drugs and have fewer side-effects, but the health implications of using these herbs on a long-term basis are still unclear. It is therefore recommended that they only be used on a short-term basis, and under the care of a qualified TCM practitioner. You should also advise your doctor of your TCM treatment.

One of the most common treatments in the Orient for symptoms of the climacteric is a phytoestrogen (plant estrogen) herb made from the root of the plant Dong Quai (known by many names such as Dang Gui and Angelica Sinensis).

Dong Quai is the most important Chinese treatment for menstrual disorders and can be effective in reducing the severity of menopausal symptoms such as:

- Hot flashes
- Irregular periods
- Spotting and flooding
- Heart palpitations
- Headaches

- Insomnia

- Anxiety
- Depression
- Fuzzy thinking
- Loss of memory, concentration, organization skills, and decision-making ability
- "Menopause Arthritis"

Dong Quai relieved my depression and fuzzy thinking; returned my memory, concentration, organization, and decision-making skills; and "turned my lights back on", within 10 days of the start of treatment.

As described in Chapter 2, I worked my way off Dong Quai over four months, after which time I experienced about three years of milder, more manageable symptoms which were not disruptive to my life.

Acupuncture/Acupressure

Acupuncture is a healing method which treats various conditions by inserting the tips of thin needles into the skin. The location of the insertion point varies, depending on the condition being treated. Every point has a specific therapeutic effect on a specific internal organ. Acupuncture is said to be able to cure specific diseases of the internal organs, and to relieve pain in bones, muscles, joints, and skin. It is usually used in conjunction with herbal prescriptions.

Acupuncture can be effective in reducing the severity of menopausal symptoms such as:

- Hot flashes
- Heavy bleeding
- Digestive problems
- Insomnia
- Mood swings

If needles in the skin don't appeal to you, acupressure follows the same principles using finger pressure, instead of needles, on the specific point.

☞ DIET

You can help to improve your menopausal experience (and your longer-term health) by changing to a diet which draws nutrients primarily from:

- Whole grains
- Legumes
- Fresh vegetables
- Fresh fruit
- Some low-fat dairy (optional)

Foods that Help Lessen Menopausal Symptoms

a) Many foods contain weak phytoestrogens (plant estrogens) which have been shown to help regulate hormones and reduce the severity of menopausal symptoms, such as:

- Hot flashes
- Night sweats
- Depression
- Mood swings

- Irritability
- Irregular periods
- Heavy bleeding

Phytoestrogens are found in abundance in soy products such as:

✓ Textured soy protein
✓ Tempeh
✓ Soy milk

✓ Roasted soy nuts
✓ Tofu

They are also found in:

✓ Whole grains (e.g., wheat, oats, corn)
✓ Other legumes (e.g., kidney beans, peas, lentils)
✓ Vegetables (e.g., fennel, celery, linseed)
✓ Fruit (e.g., apples, figs, dates, apricots)

b) *Bioflavonoids* are nutrients which are also considered effective in reducing the severity of menopausal symptoms. Bioflavonoids are non-toxic and can be found in abundance in the pulp and white rind of citrus fruits such as:

✓ Oranges, lemons, grapefruit

They are also found in:

✓ Grapes
✓ Plums
✓ Apricots
✓ Black Currants
✓ Cherries

✓ Blackberries
✓ Rose Hips
✓ Buckwheat
✓ Green Peppers
✓ Tomatoes

Foods to Avoid

a) Some foods deplete the body of valuable nutrients needed to help cope with hormonal changes. Other foods can trigger symptoms. The following foods can worsen menopausal symptoms:

✗ Alcohol
✗ Caffeine (coffee, tea, chocolate, colas)
✗ Sugar

Supplementation

a) *Vitamin E*, in the recommended dosage of 400-800 IUs/day, has been found to reduce:

- Hot flashes
- Night sweats
- Vaginal dryness

It can take up to six weeks to take effect. If you have heart disease take it in dry form, to avoid consuming oil.

b) *Evening Primrose Oil* has been found to reduce:

- Hot flashes
- Night sweats
- Breast tenderness
- Insomnia

Take it under the direction of an herbalist, naturopath, or doctor.

c) *Bioflavonoids* (e.g., citrin, hesperidin, rutin, flavones, and flavonals) within a Vitamin C supplement are recommended. Take 500 mg of Vitamin C, twice daily. (Check first with your Doctor to ensure that this does not counteract the effectiveness of drugs or treatments you may be taking.)

Eat Regularly

To maintain a more stable mood and body, eat small, nutritious meals every 2-3 hours.

☞ EXERCISE

Exercise increases the flow of oxygen to all cells in the body, including the brain.

Exercise stimulates your adrenal glands to convert the hormone androstenedione into estrogen in your body, offsetting the impact of declining levels due to menopause. Exercise also helps to regulate your hormones.

Exercise can help to reduce the menopausal symptoms of:

- Depression
- Anxiety
- Hot flashes
- Insomnia
- Joint pain
- Fatigue

Exercise can also:

- Boost optimism, energy, mood, and self-esteem
- Improve circulation
- Improve mental functioning
- Create energy
- Increase capacity for handling stress

Exercise is an important component of getting through the menopausal years. Incorporate it into your day. Be as physically active as possible.

Exercise recommendations are made under Step 7 in Chapter 8, "Improving Your Long-Term Health Prospects".

NON-DRUG SOLUTIONS TO
SOME DIFFICULT MENOPAUSAL SYMPTOMS

Physical Symptoms

Heavy Bleeding (Flooding)

This is one of the most serious problems caused by hormonal imbalance because prolonged heavy bleeding inevitably leads to iron-deficiency anemia. Iron-deficiency anemia causes debilitating fatigue, dizziness, mental confusion, and reduced immune system function. This is an urgent health problem!

Heavy bleeding is to blame for approximately 25% of all hysterectomies in North America. A hysterectomy for hormone-related heavy bleeding is unnecessary.

If you start to experience heavier or longer bleeding during menstrual periods, see your gynecologist about having the Reproductive Organ tests in the Test Checklist (see Chapter 5) to rule out disease. Also ask for the Iron-Deficiency Anemia blood tests which are listed in the Test Checklist. It is very important to keep your iron at healthy levels.

Most non-drug approaches to remedying heavy menstrual bleeding are based on avoiding the blood build-up in the endometrial (uterine) lining which occurs when menstrual periods are missed. This blood can eventually flow out through heavy bleeding or "flooding". Regulating menstrual periods will help to reduce heavy bleeding. Try the following alternatives to regulate menstrual periods.

- Consume bioflavonoids, found in citrus fruits, other fruits, and supplementation, as suggested in the "Diet" section, earlier in this chapter.

- Have acupuncture treatments.

- Take herbal progesterone under the direction of a qualified health care practitioner.

- Follow other suggestions made by a naturopath or a traditional Chinese doctor.

- If the above approaches are not effective for you, consult your gynecologist to discuss the option of having an *endometrial ablation.*

In an endometrial ablation, the lining of the endometrium (uterus) is cauterized and destroyed, and blood build-up is not supposed to occur again. It is a one hour procedure done by a medical doctor, on an outpatient basis, under general anesthetic. After this procedure, menstrual bleeding is supposed to be minimal or non-existent, and pregnancy is said to be impossible. It is a new procedure, and long-term side-effects, if any, are as yet unknown.

Expect severe pelvic cramping for about 24 hours after the ablation. Bed rest is advised for 2-3 days after the procedure. After that, return to normal activities.

I had an endometrial ablation in mid-1994. My menstrual periods after that were usually very light, just enough to allow me to continue to track my way through menopause. However, in one instance, after skipping four menstrual periods, I experienced heavy bleeding in the menstrual period which followed. This was almost "flooding", but lasted only 4-5 days. I have had annual pap smears, pelvic exams, and transvaginal ultrasounds since the ablation, and there are no indications of any adverse side-effects.

Severe iron-deficiency anemia, which I experienced as a result of prolonged, heavy bleeding prior to the ablation, and the accompanying debilitating fatigue, have been replaced by a high iron count and a high energy level. Fear of flooding, which had limited my activities for an extended period of time, became a thing of the past.

Fatigue Caused by Iron-Deficiency Anemia

If you have been experiencing prolonged, heavy bleeding, you will eventually begin to exhibit the following symptoms of Iron-Deficiency Anemia:

- Fatigue after minimal exertion
- Lethargy and weakness
- Shortness of breath
- Rapid heartbeat
- Confusion
- Difficulty concentrating
- Dizziness

Watch for this. It can sneak up on you and be passed off as stress, overwork, or "aging". If you have any of these symptoms, see your doctor immediately and have your blood levels of hemoglobin and ferritin checked to confirm the diagnosis and determine the severity of your condition. Take dietary action to reverse iron-deficiency anemia.

To increase iron in the blood and reverse iron-deficiency anemia:

- Eat iron-rich food
  - ✓ Red meat, especially liver
  - ✓ Oysters, clams
  - ✓ Legumes (chickpeas, lentils, beans)
  - ✓ Iron-fortified grains
  - ✓ Prunes, raisins, prune juice
  - ✓ Brown rice
  - ✓ Seaweed
  - ✓ Yellow, orange, red, green vegetables

- Enhance absorption with
  - ✓ Vitamin C-rich foods (e.g., fruit)

- Take iron-rich herbs
  - ✓ Dandelion leaf, dandelion root
  - ✓ Yellow dock root

- Take iron supplements
  - ✓ "Floradix Formula Herbal Iron Extract"
  - ✓ Iron tablets (refer to your doctor or pharmacist)

- Avoid iron-depleting foods
  - ✗ Alcohol
  - ✗ Carbonated drinks
  - ✗ Aspirin
  - ✗ Caffeine (coffee, tea, chocolate, colas)
  - ✗ Too much dairy

Hot Flashes/Night Sweats

Approximately 80% of North American women and almost no Japanese or Chinese women experience this symptom. Hot flashes and night sweats are thought to be caused by a sharp drop in estrogen. If you experience these often, your estrogen is probably volatile.

To lessen the severity and frequency of hot flashes and night sweats:

- Eat effectively (see "Diet" section)
  - ✓ Small, nutritious meals every 2-3 hours

        ✔ Soy products
        ✔ Whole grains (wheat, oats, corn)
        ✔ Other Legumes (beans, peas, lentils)
        ✔ Vegetables (fennel, celery, linseed)
        ✔ Fruit (apples, figs, dates, apricots)
        ✔ Foods with bioflavonoids

- Exercise   ✔ Daily, if possible

- Keep cool   ✔ Drink ice water often.
        ✔ Do not overdress.
        ✔ Keep thermostats down.

- Reduce stress   ✔ Learn relaxation techniques.

- Take supplements   ✔ Vitamin E, 400-800 IUs/day
        ✔ Bioflavonoids in a 500 mg Vitamin C tablet, twice daily
        ✔ Evening Primrose Oil

- Have acupuncture or acupressure   ✔

- Take herbs   ✔ Black Cohosh
        ✔ Siberian Ginseng (eleutherococcus)
        ✔ Dong Quai (takes 1-2 wks to take effect)
        ✔ Vitex

- Avoid symptom-causing   ✗ Alcohol (especially red wine)
        ✗ Sugar
        ✗ Caffeine (coffee, tea, chocolate, colas)
        ✗ Tobacco
        ✗ Stress
        ✗ Emotional upset

Intellectual and Emotional Symptoms

Intellectual and emotional symptoms cannot be truly understood unless they have been experienced. They are the major reason why many women resort to HRT.

Depression, anxiety, short-term memory loss, loss of ability to concentrate and to make decisions, can all result from hormonal changes and imbalances. These are frightening symptoms which make a woman weak and vulnerable.

It is important to do what you can to minimize the impact of these temporary symptoms on your life and your future. Find two or three people you can trust to confide in and rely on for non-judgemental, positive reinforcement and level-headed support during these difficult years. Seek their counsel and assistance for decisions.

Remember, although these symptoms may persist for a couple of years, they will *not last forever.* The strengths and abilities you had come to rely on will return. You will be yourself again. Lean on your supporters, and banish from your life anyone who implies that your symptoms are caused by personal weakness and/or failure of your coping skills.

To lessen the severity of all intellectual and emotional symptoms:

- Eat effectively
  (see "Diet" section)
  - ✓ Small, nutritious meals every 2-3 hours
  - ✓ Soy products
  - ✓ Whole grains (wheat, oats, corn)
  - ✓ Other Legumes (beans, peas, lentils)
  - ✓ Vegetables (fennel, celery, linseed)
  - ✓ Fruit (apples, figs, dates, apricots)
  - ✓ Foods with bioflavonoids
  - ✓ Some low-fat dairy products

- Exercise
  - ✓ Daily, if possible - aerobic exercise that gets your heart pumping

Further suggestions for each individual symptom are outlined below.

Depression

For the majority of women, depression during the climacteric is caused by:

a) Declining and/or out-of-balance hormone levels

b) Discouragement and anger at feeling ill and out of control of their bodies and lives for a long time - it is the sense of helplessness and hopelessness

Depression caused by hormonal imbalance can be severe and frightening. It is quite different from the sad or melancholy feeling many women have upon realizing that their child-bearing years are over, or that their babies have grown up, or that their parents' health is failing. It is not something anyone can "snap out of", or control.

Nor can any amount of costly professional counselling have an impact on this kind of depression. More likely, counselling will be given the credit for something that happens naturally, with time. Once hormones stabilize, and a woman's body has adapted to her post-menopausal hormone levels, depression usually lifts and a feeling of well-being returns. In the meantime, lean on your two or three supporters to talk your way through this difficult time.

To lessen the severity of depression:

- Take supplements
  - ✓ Vitamin B complex - 50 mg/day
  - ✓ Bioflavonoids in a 500 mg Vitamin C tablet, twice daily

- Have acupuncture or acupressure
  - ✓

- Take herbs
  - ✓ Dandelion root tea
  - ✓ Siberian Ginseng (eleutherococcus)
  - ✓ Dong Quai (takes 1-2 wks to take effect)

- Avoid symptom-causing
  - ✗ Alcohol
  - ✗ Caffeine (coffee, tea, chocolate, colas)
  - ✗ Sugar
  - ✗ White flour

Anxiety

Anxiety manifests itself in a number of ways, such as:

a)   Your body trembles from inside out. You feel "wired" all the time.

b)   You fret and feel weak and vulnerable.

Try to express your fears and anxieties confidentially to your two or three supporters. Once your hormones settle at post-menopausal levels, the trembling and anxieties will end, and a sense of calm and confidence will take their place.

To lessen anxiety:

- Take supplements
  - ✓ Bioflavonoids in a 500 mg Vitamin C tablet, twice daily

- Have acupuncture or acupressure
  - ✓

- Take herbs
  - ✓ Stinging Nettle
  - ✓ Valerian Root tea - use no more than 3 times a week
  - ✓ Dong Quai (takes 1-2 wks to take effect)

- Avoid symptom-causing
  - ✗ Alcohol
  - ✗ Caffeine (coffee, tea, chocolate, colas)
  - ✗ Sugar

Loss of Short-Term Memory, Concentration, Decision-Making Ability

Intellectual symptoms are some of the most difficult symptoms to combat without drugs. Depending on your responsibilities in life, these symptoms can lead to serious consequences. As your menstrual periods come to an end, these symptoms should disappear. Mine did.

To lessen the impact of temporary loss of memory, concentration, & decision-making ability:

• Change some habits (temporarily)	✓ Make "to do" lists.
	✓ Make detailed notes of conversations or events.
	✓ Tape-record conversations.
	✓ Focus on one task at a time.
	✓ Postpone decisions or consult with sensible, trustworthy people.
• Eat effectively	✓ Foods with Vitamin B12 (oats, wheat, bran, dairy)
• Take supplements	✓ Vitamin B12 - 50 mcg/day
• Have acupuncture or acupressure	✓
• Take herbs	✓ Garden Sage
	✓ Siberian Ginseng (eleutherococcus)
	✓ Dong Quai (takes 1-2 wks to take effect)
	✓ Ginkgo Biloba
• Avoid symptom-causing	✗ Alcohol
	✗ Sugar

CHAPTER CONCLUSION

Getting through the menopausal years without drugs can be a major challenge for many women. But since most symptoms of menopause are temporary, temporary help is all that is really needed. Hopefully, some of the non-drug therapies suggested in this chapter will reduce your symptoms to a manageable level.

The longer-term challenge for all women is to protect their heart and bones from deteriorating health associated with lower post-menopause hormone levels. The final two chapters in this book, Chapter 8, "Improving Your Long-Term Health Prospects", and Chapter 9, "Osteoporosis & Bone Fracture" provide a detailed approach to doing just that, without drugs.

OTHER RECOMMENDED READING

Title:	***Natural Medicine for Menopause and Beyond***
Author:	Paula Maas, Susan E. Brown and Nancy Bruning
Published:	1997
Publisher:	Dell Publishing
ISBN:	0-440-50703-0

8
IMPROVING YOUR LONG-TERM HEALTH PROSPECTS

The major health risks facing many North American women, from menopause onward, are cardiovascular disease (heart & arteries), osteoporosis, and cancer. In my opinion, the reason for this is that many North American women have been laying the groundwork for ill-health for several decades, by eating the unhealthy standard North American diet; leading inactive, sedentary lives; and for some, engaging in destructive lifestyle habits such as smoking.

Pre-Menopause Hormone Levels Protect Women from the Consequences of Bad Habits

Prior to menopause, a woman's natural hormone levels are considered to protect her heart and bones from the ravages of unhealthy eating and lifestyle habits. Estrogen and progesterone, of which the main purpose is to keep the female body in a state of readiness for reproduction, have the happy side benefits of contributing towards maintaining the strength of a woman's heart and bones during her reproductive years.

Men do not enjoy the same hormonal advantages. Therefore, the standard North American diet and unhealthy lifestyle negatively affect their hearts at an earlier age. In the case of osteoporosis, men do not suffer the same incidence as women because their larger body size and weight build denser bones.

Post-Menopausal Cause and Effect

Be sure to get the cause and effect straight. In my opinion, it is not because of declining hormone levels that many women experience an increase in cardiovascular disease and osteoporosis after menopause. It is because of decades of destructive diet, physical inactivity, and poor lifestyle habits, against which lower post-menopausal hormone levels cannot provide protection.

Post-Menopausal HRT Attempts to Protect Women from the Consequences of Bad Habits

Also in my opinion, for the most part, long-term hormone replacement therapy (HRT) is a drug regimen which attempts to protect women from the consequences bad habits, after their own natural hormonal protection ends. Unfortunately,

1.   *Hormone drugs do not guarantee cardiovascular good health or strong bones.*

and

2.   *The side-effects of hormone drugs can range from troublesome to life-threatening.*

Eat Your Way to Better Health

The foods you eat play an enormous role in determining your health and the illnesses from which you will suffer in your lifetime. High consumption of foods of animal origin (i.e., meat, fish, fowl, eggs, dairy) and fat are now considered to be major culprits in the development of human disease.

The standard North American diet is high in foods of animal origin and fat; and low in whole grains, legumes, fresh vegetables, and fresh fruit. This is why the incidence of cardiovascular disease, osteoporosis, cancer, and other illnesses is reaching frightening levels in North America. Don't believe anyone who tells you that this is just what happens in an aging population.

The American Dietetic Association's position paper on vegetarian diets provides substantial evidence that a diet low in foods of animal origin and fat can play an important role in halting and reversing cardiovascular disease, and in lowering the incidence of some forms of cancer (e.g., lung, colon, rectal, breast).[1]

A low-fat, lacto-ovo-vegetarian diet ("lacto" includes dairy products; "ovo" includes eggs; no other animal foods are consumed) has also been shown to lower the incidence of osteoporosis.[2]

Step 6, in this chapter, will suggest ways for you to make beneficial changes to your diet and eat your way to better health.

Exercise Your Way to Better Health

An inactive, sedentary, lifestyle also contributes to an increase in the risk of many illnesses, including cardiovascular disease, osteoporosis, and cancer.

Step 7, in this chapter, will suggest ways for you to make beneficial changes to your physical activities and exercise your way to better health.

Your Fate is not Sealed

We are not necessarily genetically doomed to suffer the same ailments, and to die from the same diseases, as our parents. Diet, physical activity, and lifestyle habits, which we often copy from our parents, strongly impact on our health and longevity. Our genes alone do not seal our fate.

The use of HRT is partially based on that genetic theory. Doctors too often prescribe hormone drugs to a woman because one of her parents has suffered from heart disease or osteoporosis.

For many women, a proper diet, an active lifestyle, and healthy habits will help protect against these dread diseases. This natural approach also has the positive side-effect of reducing cancer risk, not increasing it, as hormone drugs may.

Live and Enjoy Long Decades Ahead

Information provided in this chapter will be of great importance to your ability to really live and enjoy long decades ahead, without drugs. It will help you to establish a diet and exercise plan to improve your long-term health prospects. The same program may also be effective in lessening the severity of your menopausal symptoms.

STEP 6: *Start the Process of Changing to a Healthier Diet.*

A low-fat diet which draws nutrients primarily from the following five food groups is recommended:

- Whole grains
- Legumes
- Fresh vegetables
- Fresh fruit
- Some low-fat dairy (optional)

This advice is echoed by more and more researchers, as they make new discoveries about the power of different plant foods, and by doctors who take the time to analyze and educate themselves in this growing field of health care through nutrition.

Within the five food groups, it is recommended that you consume daily servings as outlined in the box on the next page.

The wide range of recommended servings reflects the wide range of sizes and activity levels of individuals. In general, a 100 lb woman with an inactive lifestyle, requires fewer servings to meet her body's nutritional and caloric needs, than an active 200 lb man.

Recommended Daily Consumption

	One Serving Equals
• 5-12 servings of whole grains	½ cup cooked rice/pasta/cereal ½ bagel/pita/bun 1 slice bread
• 2-3 servings of legumes	½ cup cooked dried beans/peas/ lentils/chickpeas 8 oz /1 cup soy milk 100gms/4oz /½ cup tofu
• 3-5 servings of fresh vegetables (Include a wide variety of colours. To cook vegetables, steam lightly or bake, for best nutritional value.)	1 medium size whole vegetable 1 cup salad 1 cup raw vegetable ½ cup cooked vegetable ¾ cup vegetable juice
• 3-5 servings of fresh fruit (Include a wide variety.)	1 medium size whole fresh fruit ½ cup cooked fruit ¾ cup fruit juice
• 1-2 servings of low-fat dairy (optional)	1 cup skim milk ¾ cup low-fat yogurt 50 gms/ 1½ oz low-fat cheese

---

SIX GOALS FOR A HEALTHIER DIET

By following the above dietary plan, and reducing your consumption of fat and cholesterol, you will be well on your way to accomplishing the six goals for a healthier diet, which are listed below. Accomplishing these six goals will reduce your risk of cardiovascular disease, osteoporosis, and cancer, and can lessen the severity of menopausal symptoms.

The six goals for a healthier diet are:

☞ **Reduce Fat Consumption**

☞ **Reduce Cholesterol Consumption**

☞ **Reduce Animal Protein Consumption**

☞ **Increase Anti-Oxidant Consumption**

☞ **Increase Fibre Consumption**

☞ **Increase Calcium Consumption**

The remainder of this chapter provides detailed information to show you how to accomplish the six goals for a healthier diet. Accomplishing these six goals will contribute greatly to your ability to get through menopause and enjoy a longer, healthier life, without drugs.

Take your time incorporating these changes into your diet. Dietary changes cannot happen overnight, especially if they affect other family members.

☞ Reduce Fat Consumption

On average, North Americans get about 34% of the day's calories from fat.[3] This is an average, which means that fat consumption for many people is much higher. Dietary fat has been implicated in most disease-caused deaths in North America today. And although it is difficult to isolate any one causal factor in a disease, research generally points to reducing fat in our diets as a healthy thing to do.

Both the Canadian Heart and Stroke Foundation and the American Heart Association consider 30% or less of the day's calories to be a healthier level of fat consumption. But many health practitioners, especially those in the forefront of cardiovascular and cancer research, advise that the number should be somewhat lower for the general population, and much lower for individuals already suffering from, or at high risk for, fat-related diseases.

Dr. Dean Ornish, in his book *Dr. Dean Ornish's Program for Reversing Heart Disease*, provides a well-known program for reversing and preventing cardiovascular disease through diet and lifestyle. His cardiovascular disease reversal diet has less than 10% fat content. His program also addresses high blood pressure, osteoporosis, and colon, breast, ovarian, and prostate cancers. It is appropriate for anyone wishing to reduce her or his risk of developing those diseases.

Title:	***Dr. Dean Ornish's Program for Reversing Heart Disease***
Author:	Dean Ornish, M.D.
Published:	1996
Publisher:	Ballantine Books
ISBN:	0-8041-1038-7

A Little Bit About Fat

One gram of fat has 9 calories. This compares with 4 calories per gram in each of carbohydrates and protein. Reducing fat in your diet will increase hunger, as your body seeks to replace all those calories. You can start to eat your way to better health, by replacing the fat calories with calories from a wide variety of nutritious, low-fat foods.

Fat is found in most foods, but in general, foods of plant origin contain substantially less fat, as a percent of calories, than foods of animal origin. A general categorization is provided in the table below.

General Fat Content of Food Groups

- Fresh fruit, fresh vegetables, and legumes (e.g., green peas, split peas, lentils, kidney beans, navy beans) contain less than 10% fat (with the exception of avocados and olives which are about 70-90% fat).

- Most whole grains (e.g., breads, cereals, pasta, rice) contain less than 10% fat.

- Fish contains 10%-20% fat, if not cooked with oil or butter.

- Fowl contains 20%-40% fat if cooked without skin, oil, or butter.

- Beef, lamb, and pork contain 20%-80% fat, depending on the type and cut.

- Most dairy products (e.g., milks, creams, cheeses) contain 40%-90% fat (except low-fat products).

- Most cakes, cookies, and pastries contain up to 60% fat.

- Nuts (including peanut butter) contain more than 70% fat.

- All oils, butter, lard, and most margarines are 100% fat.

Fats are of two different types: saturated and unsaturated.

Saturated fats are the most deadly for your heart and arteries and should be minimized in your diet. Saturated fats are used by the liver to manufacture cholesterol, especially the "bad" LDL cholesterol, which most contributes to cardiovascular disease.

Saturated fats are highest in foods of animal origin. Plant foods are low in saturated fats, with the exception of some, such as, olives, nuts, seeds, coconut, chocolate. Saturated fats are solid at room temperature and are usually found in high amounts in baked goods and fried foods.

Examples of oils which are high in saturated fat are butter, coconut oil, shortening, and palm oil.

Unsaturated fats (polyunsaturated and monounsaturated) are essential for good health, as long as they are consumed primarily as part of the make-up of the foods you eat. It is not healthy to consume large quantities of these fats in pure oil form (e.g., in salad dressings or in cooking).

The oils with the lowest saturated fat and the highest unsaturated fat content are olive and canola (lowest).

The following book provides a good discussion of fats and cholesterol and how they affect the human body. It also lists the calories, fat grams, saturated fat grams, cholesterol milligrams, and percentage fat content for 700 pages of food items.

Title:	***The NutriBase Guide to Fat & Cholesterol in Your Food***
Author:	Dr. Art Ulene
Published:	1995
Publisher:	Avery Publishing Group
ISBN:	0-89529-633-0

How Much Fat is Right for You?

For health purposes, fat must be measured as a percent of food calories, not as a percent of food weight.

Fat requirement varies by individual, depending on age, weight, activity level, and current disease status. To determine how much fat is right for you, you must:

1. *Know how many food calories you consume daily*

2. *Decide what percentage of calories you wish to consume in the form of fat*

3. *Calculate your desired daily fat limit*

The remainder of this section about fat will provide you with enough knowledge to select appropriate foods so that you can stay within your chosen fat consumption limit.

1. *Know how many food calories you consume daily*

Count your actual daily calorie intake for a few days. Use the nutritional information on packaged goods you buy, and *The NutriBase Guide to Fat & Cholesterol in Your Food* or a similar reference book, for fresh foods. (calories = energy in food labels)

Insert the number of food calories you consume daily, on this line: _____ **(1)**

2. *Decide what percentage of calories you wish to consume in the form of fat*

Using the following guidelines, decide how much fat you wish to consume, as a percentage of your total calorie consumption.

- The Canadian Heart and Stroke Foundation and the American Heart Association recommend that fat intake be *30%* or less of calories.

- Health practitioners in the specialties of cancer and cardiovascular disease generally recommend that fat intake be no more than *20%* of calories.

- The Canadian Women's Health Initiative recommends no more than *15%* of calories from fat.

- Both Dr. Dean Ornish, in his program for reversing heart disease without drugs, surgery, or other medical intervention, and Dr. John McDougall in his program for a healthy heart recommend that fat intake be less than *10%* of calories.

Insert the percentage of calories you wish to eat in the form of fat, here:_____% (**2**)

3. *Calculate your desired daily fat limit*

Estimate the maximum number of grams of fat you would like to consume each day, by filling in the blanks in the formula provided after the example below. Insert your estimated daily calorie consumption from (**1**) above, and your desired daily fat percentage from (**2**) above.

Example:

If you eat about 1,850 calories a day and wish to restrict the fat in your diet to 20% of calories, you must limit your daily fat consumption to 41 grams, as calculated below.

$$\underset{\text{(calories)}}{1,850} \times \underset{\text{(\%)}}{20\%} = \underset{\text{(fat calories)}}{370} \div 9^* = \underset{\text{(rounded)}}{41} \text{ grams}$$

Your Calculation:

$$\underset{\text{(calories)}}{\rule{2cm}{0.4pt}} \times \underset{\text{(\%)}}{\rule{1.5cm}{0.4pt}} = \underset{\text{(fat calories)}}{\rule{1.5cm}{0.4pt}} \div 9^* = \underset{\text{(rounded)}}{\rule{1cm}{0.4pt}} \text{ grams}$$

*1 gram of fat = 9 calories. Therefore, the number of fat calories must be divided by 9 to determine the number of grams of fat to which you wish to limit yourself.

How to Figure Out the Percentage Fat Content in Different Foods

There are two places to look to determine the percentage of fat in foods.

a) For *non-packaged goods*, determine the fat content as a percentage of calories by using *The NutriBase Guide to Fat & Cholesterol in Your Food*, or a similar reference.

b) For *packaged goods*, beware! A calculation is usually necessary. Read nutritional information on food packages and calculate fat content as a percentage of calories by multiplying the number of fat grams by 9, and dividing the result by the number of calories. (There are 9 calories in one gram of fat.)

The milk example in the box below demonstrates how to calculate fat as a percentage of calories. The calorie and fat numbers come from nutritional information on the packaging.

1 cup/250 ml milk			
Skim milk	Energy/Calories	91	Percentage fat content equals:
	Fat	0.5 grams	$(0.5 \times 9) \div 91 = 4.9\%$ fat
1% milk	Energy/Calories	108	Percentage fat content equals:
	Fat	2.7 grams	$(2.7 \times 9) \div 108 = 22.5\%$ fat
2% milk	Energy/Calories	129	Percentage fat content equals:
	Fat	5.0 grams	$(5.0 \times 9) \div 129 = 34.9\%$ fat
Whole milk	Energy/Calories	157	Percentage fat content equals:
	Fat	8.6 grams	$(8.6 \times 9) \div 157 = 49.3\%$ fat

The 2% in 2% milk, for example, refers to the fat content as a percentage of weight. This is a meaningless number which implies that 2% milk is relatively low fat, when the fat content is actually 34.9% of calories.

Don't be Fooled by Misleading Claims of Fat Content!!

Don't be fooled by what borders on misleading advertising. Manufacturers of high-fat products often state fat content as a percentage of weight instead of as a percentage of calories. They do not specifically say percentage of weight, they just say percentage. Calories and weight are not the same. They are not comparable. Weight is irrelevant.

Manufacturers and retailers often count on lack of public knowledge, to sell high-fat products. They know that people are concerned about fat consumption. They also know that most people are not yet well enough informed about fat consumption to know the difference between weight and calories. Products are often sold using a low-fat feature, when they are not low-fat in terms of your health.

For example, on a package of chicken bacon in my local grocery store, the large print shouts: *"Contains less than 17% fat."* Anyone wishing to keep fat intake to less than 20 % of calories might buy that, thinking they were staying within their chosen limit. The nutritional information provided on the package reads as follows:

Per 100 grams weight	
Energy	206 calories
Protein	12.5 grams
Fat	*16.9 grams*

From the nutritional information on the package, it is apparent that 16.9 grams of fat is the amount of fat per 100 grams of weight. Therefore, the claim on the package refers to fat content which is less than 17% of weight, not calories. From the same nutritional information, it can be determined that this chicken bacon provides 73.8% of calories in the form of fat, as calculated below.

16.9 grams of fat $\times$ 9 = 152.1 fat calories $\div$ 206 calories = *73.8% of calories!*

In Summary, to Manage Your Fat Consumption

✓ Learn the fat content of non-packaged foods you eat, in terms of *percentage of calories.*

✓ Ignore advertising claims and do your own percentage fat calculation for packaged foods.

✓ Replace fat calories with a wide variety of nutritious, low-fat foods.

☞ Reduce Cholesterol Consumption

Many people in North America should take action to reduce their Total Cholesterol level and their HDL Ratio. Refer to your cholesterol test results and Chapter 6, to determine whether you should too.

Excess dietary cholesterol, especially the "bad" LDL cholesterol, is considered to be a major contributor to heart disease and stroke. Cholesterol can clog up the arteries through which oxygen-rich blood flows to the heart and brain.

For most people, the liver manufactures all the cholesterol their body needs, independent of diet. The body's cholesterol level is increased through diet in the following two ways:

1. By eating cholesterol directly in foods. Cholesterol is found only in foods of animal origin. There is no cholesterol in foods of plant origin.

2. By eating saturated fats. Saturated fats are converted into cholesterol by the liver. Saturated fats are highest in foods of animal origin, but are also in foods of plant origin.

Make note that a "no cholesterol" claim for a food is only half the story. If a food has no cholesterol but does have saturated fat, that food will raise the body's cholesterol level just as if cholesterol were being eaten.

The American Heart Association recommends daily cholesterol consumption of less than 300 milligrams.

A Healthy Total Cholesterol Level

Dr. Dean Ornish and Dr. John McDougall both recommend maintenance of a Total Cholesterol blood level of 150 mg/dl or lower (3.9 mmol/l in Canadian terms) to prevent or reverse cardiovascular disease. If you maintain a Total Cholesterol blood count at or below this level, they consider it very unlikely that you will become a victim of heart disease. You certainly won't need HRT to protect you from cardiovascular disease.

A Healthy HDL Ratio

Dr. William Castelli, medical director of the Framingham, Massachusetts Cardiovascular Institute, considers the HDL Ratio to be a better predictor of risk of cardiovascular disease than Total Cholesterol. He considers a ratio of 4.0 or less to be healthy.[4]

Some Research Findings

- Vitamin E has been shown to reduce cholesterol and the incidence of cardiovascular disease.[5-7] Dr. McDougall, in his book, suggests a daily dosage of 400 IUs. If you have cardiovascular disease, take it in "dry form" to avoid consuming oil.

What To Do if Your Total Cholesterol and HDL Ratio are Too High

If your medical test results show that your Total Cholesterol and HDL Ratio are too high:

- Talk to your doctor about trying to manage the reduction of both levels through diet and lifestyle changes, before resorting to drugs.

- Educate yourself in non-drug methods of managing your heart health. *Dr. Dean Ornish's Program for Reversing Heart Disease* will provide ample information on how to do this, naturally.

- Educate yourself about what foods are high in cholesterol and saturated fats. *The NutriBase Guide to Fat & Cholesterol in Your Food* will provide this information. Also read the nutritional information provided on the packages of foods you buy.

- Take the following immediate action, at least to some degree, until you have developed a long-term heart health plan with your health practitioner.

  a) Minimize your consumption of cholesterol by minimizing your consumption of oils and foods of animal origin (i.e., meat, fish, fowl, eggs, dairy).

  b) Minimize saturated fats in your diet.

  c) Increase the amount of fresh fruit, fresh vegetables, and whole grains you eat.

  d) Stop consuming caffeine (e.g., coffee, tea, chocolate, colas), sugar, and food additives.

  e) Stop smoking.

  f) Take 400 mg of dry form (non-oil) Vitamin E, daily.

☞ Reduce Animal Protein Consumption

Protein is called an "energy nutrient" because it provides calories, or energy, to the body.

$$1 \text{ gram of protein} = 4 \text{ calories}$$

Protein is made up of 22 different amino acids, all of which are necessary for good health. 13 of the amino acids are made by the body. The rest, called "essential amino acids", must be obtained through food.

Complete vs. Incomplete Proteins

Complete proteins contain all 22 kinds of amino acids and are found primarily in foods of animal origin (i.e., meat, fish, fowl, eggs, dairy). Complete proteins are also found in soy milk, soy beans, and some grains.

Incomplete proteins do not contain all "essential amino acids", and are found in grains, legumes (e.g., kidney beans, lima beans, chickpeas, lentils), seeds, and nuts. The body requires *complete* proteins for good health. To create a complete protein from plant foods, a grain and a legume must be eaten on the same day.

Acid-Producing vs. Alkaline Proteins

Some proteins are acid-producing proteins and some are alkaline proteins.

Acid-producing proteins have been shown to cause an increase in the loss of calcium from the body, through the urine.[8] *Non-dairy* foods of animal origin are known to contain acid-producing protein, but there is a lack of consensus as to the type of protein found in dairy products.

Most plant foods contain alkaline proteins and are known to reduce the acidity of the urine, thereby reducing urinary calcium excretion.[9] (Refer to Chapter 9, "Osteoporosis & Bone Fracture", for further details.)

Some Research Findings

Osteoporosis is a disease characterized by porous and fragile bones which are vulnerable to easy fracture. Excess consumption of protein from foods of animal origin is now being studied as possibly one of the primary factors leading to the development of osteoporosis.

- Urinary calcium excretion has been shown to increase with the consumption of *non-dairy* foods of animal origin, and to decrease with the consumption of vegetables and fruits.[10]

- Lacto-Ovo-Vegetarians (consume dairy products and eggs; but do not eat meat, fish, or fowl) experience a much lower incidence of bone loss in the later years than meat-eaters, and are less prone to osteoporosis.[11]

- In a large study of older Caucasian women, meat-eaters lost 35% of their bone mass between ages 50-89; whereas, lacto-vegetarians lost only 18%.[12]

Chapter 9, "Osteoporosis & Bone Fracture", reviews the findings and issues surrounding causes and prevention of osteoporosis.

How Much Protein is Right for You?

On average, North Americans consume 2-3 times their daily protein requirement. Protein requirement varies by individual depending on age, body size, and health. For a healthy adult over 19 years of age, calculate your daily protein requirement by multiplying your weight times 0.36. Fill in the blanks below.

$$\underline{\hspace{3cm}} \text{ lbs.} \quad \times \quad 0.36 \quad = \quad \underline{\hspace{2cm}} \text{ grams per day}$$

(your weight)   (rounded)

It is important to have a good portion of your daily protein requirement at the start of your day, for energy. A large bowl of multi-grain cereal (6-8 grams of protein) in 1 cup of soy milk (4 grams of protein), or 1 cup of skim milk (8-9 grams of protein), will provide most people with about 25% of their daily protein requirement.

The correct amount of protein is important for normal body function and for the maintenance of body tissues but, more is not better.

How do You Know How Much Protein You are Eating?

- Nutritional information on packaged foods usually states protein content.

- A general approximation of the amounts of protein found in different food groups is provided in the table below. Protein amounts vary by individual food item within each group.

- Nuts and seeds are high in protein, but also very high in saturated fats, and have not been included in this list.

Protein Table		
Animal Origin Foods	**Quantity**	**Protein (gms)**
Beef/Chicken/Turkey	4 oz	25-35
Fish		
• Various	4 oz	20-30
• Fish stick	1	5
Processed Meats		
• hot dog	1	7
• bologna	1 slice	3
• salami	4 oz	20
Dairy		
• milk/yogurt	1 cup	8-12
• cottage cheese	1 cup	25-30
• other cheeses	1 oz	4-9
Egg	1	6
Plant Origin Foods		
Legumes/Beans		
• lima, lentils, , white, navy, kidney & black beans, chickpeas, soybeans	1 cup - cooked	10-15
• soy milk	1 cup	8
• tofu	3.5 oz	8
Grains		
• pita - whole wheat	1	6
• rye/whole wheat bread	1 slice	2
• oatmeal cereal	1 cup - cooked	6
• pasta	1 cup	5
• rice - brown, wild	1 cup - cooked	5-6
• barley	1 cup - cooked	5
Vegetables		
• green peas	1 cup	8
• broccoli, brussels sprouts, yams corn, winter squash, carrots	1 cup	2-5
Fruit		
• fresh, canned, frozen, juice, dried	1 cup/ 1 fruit	5-6

☞ Increase Anti-Oxidant Consumption

Anti-oxidants are disease-fighting nutrients which help to protect our bodies from the negative impact of free-radicals. Anti-oxidants slow the body's aging process and can significantly reduce the risk of contracting major diseases.

Anti-oxidants are found primarily in fruit, vegetables, and whole grains. At least 100 anti-oxidants have been discovered and are currently under study. Because different foods contain different anti-oxidants, it is important to eat a wide variety of fruit, vegetables, and whole grains, in order to derive the most health benefits. It is recommended that you eat 6-10 servings of fresh fruit & vegetables, and 5-12 servings of whole grains, each day.

Free-radicals are destructive molecules within the human body. They speed the aging process and lead to disease development, by destroying healthy cells.

Free-radicals form as a result of damage to the body. They attack our healthy cells in huge numbers every day. When they form and attack healthy cells at a faster rate than the body can repair itself, disease development is more likely. The best way to minimize the destructive impact of free-radicals is to avoid those things which create them, and to eat lots of anti-oxidants.

Free-radicals can be created by many things, such as, stress, pollution, chemicals, smoking, sunlight, food additives & preservatives, radiation, fat, cholesterol, alcohol, and poor diet.

Free-radicals are kept in check by anti-oxidants. Researchers now consider anti-oxidants to have the potential to prevent diseases through diet.

The most common anti-oxidants found in food and the ones we currently know best are:

Vitamin C

Vitamin E

Vitamin A (Beta-Carotene)

Vitamin C

Vitamin C is a powerful anti-oxidant which helps to strengthen the body's immune system. It is important for the growth and repair of body tissue cells, blood vessels, bones, teeth, and gums. The human body does not make its own Vitamin C. It must be obtained from food. Vitamin C is used up more rapidly by the body during times of stress, disease, fever, and toxic exposure (e.g., smoking). Its absorption in the body is enhanced when taken with bioflavonoids.

More Facts About Vitamin C

- fights bacterial and viral infections
- protects against heart disease
- counteracts cancer-causing substances
- reduces effects of many allergy-causing substances

Best Vitamin C Food Sources

- citrus fruit
- berries
- green vegetables
- leafy vegetables
- tomatoes
- cauliflower
- peppers

Recommended Vitamin C plus Bioflavonoid Supplement

- 500 mg, twice daily (double during times of stress or infection)

Vitamin E

Vitamin E is a strong defender of the body from free-radical damage. Vitamin E provides protection for the heart and blood vessels. Vegetarians tend to have higher levels of Vitamin E in the bloodstream than non-vegetarians. Vitamin E assists the body's immune system in fighting viral infections.

More Facts About Vitamin E

- slows cellular aging
- lowers cholesterol
- prevents and dissolves blood clots
- lowers blood pressure
- protects against the formation of cataracts
- in ointment form on skin, promotes healing of burned tissue, skin ulcers, and abrasions; lessens formation of scars
- reduces PMS and Menopause symptoms

Best Vitamin E Food Sources

- whole wheat
- brown rice
- millet
- cucumber
- kale

Recommended Vitamin E Supplement

- 200-400 IUs/day (for heart disease, take in dry form to avoid consuming oil)
- 400-800 IUs/day for menopausal women

Vitamin A (Beta-Carotene)

Vitamin A helps in the growth and repair of body tissues. It strengthens the body's immune system so that it is better able to fight invading bacteria and to counter the production of abnormal cells which can develop into cancer. Low Vitamin A levels put the body at risk for developing cancer.

Vitamin A is only found in foods of animal origin. Beta-Carotene is the plant source of Vitamin A which is converted to Vitamin A, once in the body. Beta-Carotene is a substance which is found at high levels in orange plant foods. Beta-Carotene has been found to be more effective if obtained through food rather than supplements.

More Facts About Vitamin A (Beta-Carotene)

- protects against cancer, especially breast, cervix, lung
- lowers risk of heart disease
- helps Vitamin C work better
- prevents night blindness
- maintains good eyesight
- builds strong teeth and bones

Best Vitamin A Food Sources

- liver
- cantaloupe
- mango
- papaya
- Nori seaweed
- carrot
- sweet potato

Recommended Vitamin A (Beta-Carotene) Supplement

- Not recommended.

A Note About Vitamin and Mineral Supplements

As the human body ages, its ability to absorb nutrients from food decreases. It is therefore important to increase your nutritional intake to offset decreased absorption. This can be done by making sure that a higher percentage of the foods you eat are nutritious (i.e., are not junk food), and perhaps, by taking supplements.

Although Vitamin C and Vitamin E supplementation are generally acknowledged as having health-enhancing value, researchers are still learning about the properties of other vitamins and minerals in supplemental form.

So far, it seems that it is best to obtain as many vitamins and minerals as possible through nutritious foods because of their natural combination of nutrients, some of which may be as yet unknown to us.

If you are currently on medication or suffering from a chronic health problem, check with your doctor *and* your pharmacist before taking supplements.

☞ Increase Fibre Consumption

Fibre is the non-digestible part of plant foods (e.g., skin of apple, husk of wheat kernel).

Fibre does not provide any nutrients or calories but performs a function in the intestines which is not yet clearly understood. Normal functioning of the intestinal tract depends on the presence of fiber. Fibre is essential for the healthy elimination of waste from the body. Fibre reduces cholesterol, and regulates blood sugar and insulin levels.

A high fibre diet has been correlated with a lower incidence of:

- colon, intestinal, and rectal cancer
- lung, breast, cervical, and prostate cancer
- cardiovascular disease
- diverticulosis
- obesity
- constipation
- hemorrhoids

The American Dietetic Association recommends daily consumption of 10 to 13 grams of dietary fibre per 1,000 calories consumed. This translates into somewhere in the range of 20-35 grams per day for most adults. Although it is important to get your daily requirement of fibre, once again, more is not better. Too much fibre can cause an increase in calcium loss.

Foods that are high in fibre also tend to be high in anti-oxidants and other vitamins and minerals. Such foods include legumes, whole grains, most fresh fruit, and some fresh vegetables. There is no fibre in foods of animal origin. The table in the box below provides the approximate fibre content of some high-fibre foods.

Fibre Table		
Legumes (cooked)	**Quantity**	**Fibre Content (gms)** [13]
• pinto beans	1 cup	8
• lima, green, navy beans	1 cup	3-4
• kidney beans, lentils	1 cup	2-3
Grains (cooked)		
• millet	1 cup	7
• wheat bran	1 cup	5
• brown rice, barley, bulgar	1 cup	2-3
• cereals: fibre content varies widely-check nutritional information on package		
Fruit		
• elderberries	1 cup	10
• blackberries	1 cup	6
• raspberries	1 cup	4
• dried figs	10	9
Vegetables		
• winter squash, carrot juice, pumpkin	1 cup	2-3

Getting Your Daily Fibre Requirement

You will have no trouble consuming your daily requirement of fibre if you:

1.   Eat 5 servings of fresh fruit or fresh vegetables, daily. Include the skins where possible. (one serving = 1 piece fruit, 1 cup raw leafy vegetable, ½ cup other fruit or vegetables, ¾ cup fruit or vegetable juice)

2.   Eat 6 servings of whole grains, cereals, or legumes daily. Make sure the grains are *whole* grains (e.g., bran or whole wheat cereal; rye, whole wheat, or oatmeal bread; brown rice). (one serving = 1 slice bread; ½ cup cooked cereal, rice, pasta, beans)

3.   Spread your fibre consumption out over the day. Eat some with each meal.

4.   Get fibre from foods, not pills or powder. Foods have other valuable nutrients too.

5.   Drink plenty of fluids to help the fibre flow painlessly through your intestines.

6.   Avoid canned or frozen fruit and vegetables. Fibre content is not as high.

☞ **Increase Calcium Consumption**

Calcium's main function is to build and maintain strong bones and teeth. Calcium also

- regulates heartbeat
- is necessary for proper blood-clotting
- improves sleep
- helps the nervous system

Calcium is an essential mineral for healthy functioning of the human body. As the human body ages, its ability to absorb calcium from food decreases.

How Much Calcium is Recommended by the "Experts"?

As part of a program to attempt to slow the rate of bone loss and reduce the risk of osteoporosis, post-menopausal women in North America are being advised by health practitioners and dairy associations to consume 1200-1500 mg of calcium a day. The National Osteoporosis Foundation in the U.S. recommends 1500 mg/day for women over 50 years of age who are not on hormone replacement therapy.

High Calcium Consumption Alone is Not the Answer

But, high calcium consumption alone is not the answer. Perhaps a high level of calcium consumption is being recommended for North American women in an attempt to reduce their risk of osteoporosis by compensating for the large calcium losses associated with their high animal protein diet.

In an osteoporosis Consensus Conference of "developed country" experts in 1993, the Conference Report recommended 1500 mg/day of calcium for post-menopausal white women. The report stated that "Requirements may differ in other ethnic groups and may be less in persons with lower protein intakes and small skeletal size." [14]

In a presentation to the National Institutes of Health, Consensus Development Conference on Optimal Calcium Intake, Dr. Robert Heaney, a well-known osteoporosis researcher, author, and member of the Board of Trustees of the National Osteoporosis Foundation said, "Differences in protein and sodium [salt] intake from one national group to another are part of the explanation why studies in different countries have shown sometimes strikingly different calcium requirements... At low sodium and protein intakes, the calcium requirement for an adult female may be as little as 450 mg/day, whereas if her intake of both nutrients is high, she may require as much as 2000 mg/day to maintain calcium balance." [15]

Controversy over Dairy Products as a Source of Calcium

As the Dairy Bureau of Canada is happy to point out in one of its brochures, "...it is a real challenge to meet your daily calcium needs without milk products." It would be difficult to eat enough plant foods in a day to obtain 1200-1500 mg of calcium. But, as discussed in the Protein section earlier in this chapter, there is controversy over the nature of the protein found in dairy products and its impact on bone health.

However, in view of the generally strong bone health of lacto-ovo-vegetarians, it seems not to be harmful to consume some calcium from dairy products, if other foods of animal origin are eliminated or minimized in the diet.

It may be more than sufficient to consume a total of 800 mg of calcium a day (including some low-fat dairy), if non-dairy animal food consumption is minimized or eliminated from the diet. (Refer to Chapter 9, "Osteoporosis & Bone Fracture" for further discussion.)

Food Sources of Calcium

The following tables provide information to help you plan a more effective calcium consumption program. These values are approximate. In general, the best sources of calcium from plant food are leafy green vegetables, legumes (beans), and whole grains.

Calcium Content of Some Plant Foods			
	mg		**mg**
1 cup soybeans (cooked)	185	1 slice rye bread	27
1 cup white beans (cooked)	170	1 slice pumpernickel bread	27
1 cup chickpeas (cooked)	85	1 slice whole wheat bread	25
3.5 oz tofu - firm/regular	225/100	1 cup soy milk	48
1 tbsp blackstrap molasses	144	1 cup turnip greens (cooked)	250
1 taco shell	109	10 oz frozen/chop'd collards	570
1 english muffin	96	1 cup kale (cooked)	175
1 cup brown rice	64	1 cup broccoli	83
1 bran muffin	57	1 leek	73
2" square cornbread	54	1 orange	52
1 whole wheat pita	49	1 cup pineapple juice	45
1 whole wheat muffin	42	1 cup tangerine juice	44
1 6" tortilla	42	1 cup orange juice	29
1 whole wheat roll	37	1 cup grape/grapefruit juice	22
1 bagel	29	1 tbsp maple syrup	21

Spinach, Swiss chard, parsley, beet greens, and rhubarb are high in calcium but also high in oxalic acid, which blocks calcium absorption. These foods should not be consumed in large quantities.

Nuts and seeds are high in calcium, but also high in fat, and should not be consumed in large quantities.

Calcium and Protein Content of Some Dairy Products		
	mg calcium	gms protein
1 cup fruit low-fat yogurt	300	10
1 cup skim milk	250	9
1 oz brick cheese	200	7
1 cup cottage cheese	150	25-30
1 oz feta cheese	140	4
1 tbsp grated parmesan cheese	69	2

Calcium Supplements

It is best to get your calcium from foods, but if you wish to take a supplement also, look for one that includes a combination of vitamins and minerals which work together to enhance calcium absorption. These are:

- calcium citrate malate (most effective type of calcium)
- magnesium (in an amount equal to half the calcium content)
- Vitamin D (400 mg/day)*
- Vitamin Bs
- copper
- manganese
- boron

Calcium is absorbed better by the body when it is taken in smaller amounts, more frequently, rather than in one large dose.

STEP 7: *Enjoy the Benefits of Moderate Exercise.*

Regular, *moderate*, aerobic, weight-bearing exercise provides enormous physical, emotional and intellectual health benefits.

Aerobic exercise increases the body's heart rate, which increases the body's intake of oxygen. Oxygen then flows to the heart, brain, muscles, and body tissues. This increases stamina and mental acuity, and strengthens the immune system.

Weight-bearing exercise puts weight on the bones, thereby increasing bone density. It also improves muscle strength, balance, and flexibility.

---

* You should not take more than 400 mg/day of supplemental Vitamin D. If Vitamin D is included in any other vitamin/mineral supplements you take, look for a calcium supplement without Vitamin D.

Examples of aerobic, weight-bearing exercise are:

- walking
- jogging
- jumping on a trampoline
- tennis

- basketball
- skiing
- bicycle riding
- squash/racquetball

Contrary to the old adage "no pain, no gain", vigorous exercise is not necessary for better health. In fact, vigorous exercise is discouraged because it risks injury. For people with cardiovascular disease, vigorous exercise can lead to sudden cardiac death; whereas, moderate exercise can protect against it. The benefits of exercise are found in moderation and regularity.

Regularity is the most important factor. It is more important for exercise to be regular than it is for it to be vigorous. Small amounts of exercise provide the greatest overall benefit and have been shown to prevent disease and prolong life. If you stop exercising, the benefits are quickly lost.

Lack of exercise increases the risk of high blood pressure, heart disease, stroke, cancer, diabetes, and more.

30 minutes a day, or 1 hour three times a week, is sufficient for major health benefits. And in this case, *more is better*. Find an exercise you enjoy and incorporate it into your day. Be as physically active as possible.

Major Benefits of Exercise - Some Research Findings

- Regular, weight-bearing exercise, is the only non-drug method shown to significantly *increase* bone density and strength after menopause. Weight-bearing exercise has been shown to add bone mass at any age, even at eighty or ninety years old. 30 minutes a day, or 1 hour three times a week, can be an effective treatment for post-menopausal bone loss.

- Women who engage in regular, weight-bearing exercise programs can either slow or reverse post-menopausal bone loss. The rate of bone mineral loss, once commenced, can be reduced by physical activity.

- No amount of supplementation, diet or drugs can offset the bone loss which occurs rapidly with immobility.

- Regular, moderate exercise decreases the risk of cardiovascular disease and restores strength to the heart muscle after a heart attack. Walking is healthy and safe for people with cardiovascular disease.

- Exercise makes the heart stronger, healthier, and larger. It also decreases the formation of blood clots and lowers blood pressure.

- Exercise can help to reduce menopausal symptoms such as depression, anxiety, hot flashes, insomnia, joint pain, and fatigue. It also boosts optimism, energy, mood, and self-esteem.

Other Benefits of Exercise

Additional benefits of exercise are listed below.

- relaxes muscles, reduces stress
- increases joint flexibility
- reduces body fat
- makes skin healthier
- reduces risk of arthritis, emphysema, hypertension
- lowers chance of developing diabetes, constipation, hemorrhoids, cancer
- improves mental functioning
- improves circulation

Best Overall Type of Exercise

- Walking briskly is the best overall type of exercise. It has the most health benefits and the lowest risk of injury or heart attack. This type of exercise strengthens your bones and muscles (including heart).

  Walk briskly. Include as many parts of your body in the activity as possible. If you do not have enough breath to talk while you walk, you are overdoing it. Slow down.

  30 minutes a day, or 1 hour three times a week, is all it takes to realize major health benefits, and *more is better*. Try to do 5 minutes of stretching before you start and 5 minutes of stretching after you finish.

- To maintain strong upper body muscles and bones, do ten push-ups a day. Start with one a day if necessary, and work up to 10 over time.

When to Exercise

Try to incorporate exercise into your regular daily activities, rather than make it one more thing on your "To Do" list. The only equipment needed is a good pair of walking shoes.

If you cannot do 30 minutes a day, or 1 hour three times a week, try to increase your daily physical activity in some way. Here are a few suggestions.

1. Where possible, walk up and down stairs instead of taking elevators or escalators.

2.   Get off the bus one stop earlier and walk a little farther on the way home from work.

3.   Leave the car at home more often and walk to do local errands.

4.   Walk for half an hour during lunch hour, before eating lunch.

When not to Exercise

- After eating, smoking or drinking
- In hot weather - this is especially bad for the heart
- In very cold weather
- During illness
- When on medication - check with your doctor first

Notes of Caution about Exercising

1.   Before starting a new exercise program, be sure to have the cardiovascular tests outlined in Chapter 5.

    Speak to your doctor about the results and confirm that the exercise program you intend to follow is healthy for you. Make sure that your heart can safely handle any planned change in activity level.

    If you currently have cardiovascular disease, there is an excellent exercise program in *Dr. Dean Ornish's Program for Reversing Heart Disease* (Chapter 12 "How to Exercise").

2.   Overdoing exercise, by pushing yourself, has the effect of depressing your immune system and lowering your resistance to illness and disease. Don't overdo it. Regular, moderate exercise is the most beneficial.

3.   Bone loss can occur in pre-menopausal women who exercise so vigorously that they miss menstrual periods. This is due to the estrogen-lowering impact of excess stress on the body.

CHAPTER SUMMARY

To eat and exercise your way to a longer, healthier life and less severe menopausal symptoms:

1. Follow a diet which draws nutrients primarily from the five food groups of:

   - Whole grains
   - Legumes
   - Fresh vegetables
   - Fresh fruit
   - Some low-fat dairy (optional)

2. Minimize consumption of fats and cholesterol.

3. Minimize or eliminate consumption of non-dairy foods of animal origin (i.e, meat, fish, fowl, eggs).

4. Keep overall protein consumption down to your daily requirement.

5. Consume lots of anti-oxidants, found primarily in whole grains, fresh vegetables, and fresh fruit.

6. Take Supplements:

   - 500 mg Vitamin C with bioflavonoids, twice daily
   - 400-800 IUs/day Vitamin E

7. Consume 10 to 13 grams of fibre per 1,000 calories consumed per day.

8. Consume at least 800 mg of calcium daily, primarily from leafy green vegetables, legumes (beans), whole grains, and some low-fat dairy (optional).

9. Enjoy regular, *moderate*, aerobic, weight-bearing exercise at least 30 minutes a day, or 1 hour three times a week. Be as physically active as possible.

References

1. The American Dietetic Association. "Position of the American Dietetic Association: Vegetarian diets." Sept. 6, 1996.

2. Marsh, A. G., Sanchez, T. V., Mickelsen, O., Keiser, J., and Mayor, G. "Cortical Bone Density of Adult Lacto-Ovo-Vegetarian and Omnivorous Women." *Journal of American Dietetic Association* 1980; 76: 148-151.

3. National Health and Nutrition Examination Surveys (NHANES III, conducted in 1990). Cited in Ernst, N. D., Sempos, C. T., Briefel, R. R., and Clark, M. "Consistency between US dietary fat intake and serum total cholesterol concentrations: the National Health and Nutrition Examination Surveys." *American Journal of Clinical Nutrition* 1997; 66(suppl): 965S-972S.

4. As advised in an article entitled "Do Your Heart Good" by Cathy Perlmutter with Susan C. Smith, Ed Slaughter, and Toby Hanlon in *Prevention* magazine, February, 1997, p. 82.

5. Qureshi, A. A. et al. "Lowering of Serum Cholesterol in Hypercholesterolemic Humans by Tocotrienols (palmvitee)." *American Journal of Clinical Nutrition* 1991; 53: 1021S-1026S.

6. Hodis, H. N. et al. "Serial Coronary Angiographic Evidence that Antioxidant Vitamin Intake Reduces Progression of Coronary Artery Atherosclerosis." *American Medical Association Journal* 1995; 273: 1849-1854.

7. Stampfer, M. J. et al. "Vitamin E Consumption and the Risk of Coronary Disease in Women." *The New England Journal of Medicine* 1993; 328: 1444-1449.

8. Hu, J-F., Zhao, X-H., Parpia, B. and Campbell, T.C. "Dietary intakes and urinary excretion of calcium and acids: a cross-sectional study of women in China." *American Journal of Clinical Nutrition* 1993; 58: 398-406.

9. Ibid.

10. Ibid.

11. Ellis, F. R., Holesh, S., and Ellis, J. W. "Incidence of Osteoporosis in Vegetarians and Omnivores." *American Journal of Clinical Nutrition* 1972; 25:555-558.

12. Sanchez, T. V., Mickelsen, O., Marsh, A. G., Garn, S. M., and Mayor, G. H. "Bone Mineral in Elderly Vegetarian and Omnivorous Females." In: Mazess R. B. ed. *Proceedings of the fourth international conference on bone measurement.* Bethesda, MD: NIAMMD 1980:94-8 (NIH publication #80-1983.) Cited in Marsh, A. G., Sanchez, T. V., Mickelsen, O., Chaffee, F. L., and Fagal, S. M. "Vegetarian Lifestyle and Bone Mineral Density." *American Journal of Clinical Nutrition* 1988; 48: 837-841.

13. Dunne, Lavon J. *Nutrition Almanac.* New York: McGraw-Hill, 1990, pp.268-307.

14. Peck, W.A., Burckhardt, P., Christiansen, C., et al. "Consensus Development Conference: Diagnosis, Prophylaxis, and Treatment of Osteoporosis." *American Journal of Medicine* 1993; 94:646-650, p.647.

15. Heaney, Robert, P. "Cofactors Influencing the Calcium Requirement-Other Nutrients." p.72. Presented at the National Institutes of Heath *Consensus Development Conference on Optimal Calcium Intake.* Available from the National Osteoporosis Foundation, U.S.A.

9

OSTEOPOROSIS & BONE FRACTURE

Many factors are suspected of contributing to the development of post-menopausal osteoporosis. But it is important to be aware that osteoporosis does not always result in bone fracture.

This chapter will discuss the definition and diagnosis of osteoporosis; review the main factors thought to affect post-menopausal bone health; and suggest a non-drug course of action for managing and protecting your bone health, starting right now.

WHAT IS OSTEOPOROSIS?

Osteoporosis was *scientifically defined*, by a group of international experts at a Consensus Conference in 1993, as "...a systemic skeletal disease characterized by *low bone mass* and *microarchitectural deterioration of bone tissue*, with a consequent increase in bone fragility and susceptibility to fracture." [1]

This scientific definition of osteoporosis is based on current understanding that the overall soundness of our bones depends on a combination of how dense they are and how well connected the underlying lattice-work of bone is. This underlying lattice-work is the bone microarchitecture to which they are referring, and provides strength to your bone structure.

Current generally available diagnostic equipment is capable of measuring bone density (bone mass), but cannot measure bone microarchitecture. Therefore, for clinical diagnostic purposes, it is the bone density measurement, alone, which is used to establish an individual's osteoporotic status.

For adult women, osteoporosis is *diagnostically defined* as, "...a value for *bone density* or bone mineral content *that is more than 2.5 standard deviations below the young adult mean*." [2] On bone densitometry reports, 2.5 standard deviations below the young adult mean is the line on the graph, below which your bone density is in the "theoretical fracture zone". (Refer to "Graph Explanation" in the "Bones" section in Chapter 6.)

Omission of the very important factor of bone microarchitecture, in the current diagnostic method, probably explains why some women with bone density readings well into the "theoretical fracture zone" (and therefore classified as severely osteoporotic) don't experience bone fracture, even after falling.[3] These women likely have a strong interconnectedness of underlying bone structure (i.e., good bone microarchitecture).

The current *diagnostic definition* of osteoporosis is one step behind the current *scientific definition* of osteoporosis, because the equipment necessary to assess bone microarchitecture is not yet widely available. Once it is, another important piece to the puzzle of predicting future bone fracture will be available.

MAIN FACTORS THOUGHT TO AFFECT POST-MENOPAUSAL BONE HEALTH

Bone structure and strength are the result of two independent activities within the bone over a lifetime: *bone formation* and *bone loss*. In women, bone is primarily formed before 30 years of age and primarily lost after menopause.[4] Therefore, your bone health after menopause will be a function of how much bone you formed before you were 30 years old, and how much you lose after menopause.

Because so many factors are considered to contribute to both bone formation and bone loss, and because all these factors interact in a complex way with each other, and differently from body to body, it is difficult to isolate any one factor to determine the degree of its individual importance to any one individual's bone health. As a result, research findings are often inconclusive, contradictory, or don't reflect what is happening to you.

Keeping this in mind, outlined below are some of the main factors generally thought to affect post-menopausal bone health.

Peak Bone Mass at Skeletal Maturity

"Peak bone mass is generally defined as the highest level of bone mass achieved as a result of normal growth… a high peak bone mass provides a larger reserve later in life."[5] The more bone a woman builds during her bone formation years; the higher her bone density will be when the bone loss, which can accompany aging, begins.

Ovarian hormones

It seems to have been generally accepted that there is a common pattern among women of "…an acceleration of bone loss that coincides…with menopause."[6] This perception is reflected in the bone densitometry graphs discussed in Chapter 6. However, research does not totally support this perception.

Accelerated bone loss has been shown, in a number of *longitudinal studies* (which followed the bone density of individual women through some of their menopausal years), to occur in the *spine*, early in the menopausal process (i.e., within the year or so prior to and the 2-3 years following the final menstrual period).[7-10]

But, in a longitudinal study of the Neck region of the *hip*, "...no significant bone loss and no relationship between rate of loss and menopausal age" was found in a group of post-menopausal women who consumed an average of 700 mg/day of calcium from diet and supplements. [11]

In the study, conducted by Bess Dawson-Hughes (a well-regarded and longstanding researcher in the field and a member of the Board of Trustees of the National Osteoporosis Foundation in the U.S.) and Susan Harris, some of the post-menopausal women lost bone density over the two years of the study; some experienced no change in bone density; and *some gained bone density*! after menopause. Therefore, in some women, changes in ovarian hormones do not have a negative impact on bone density.

Calcium Consumption

Although it is known that calcium absorption in the body declines as we age [12], there is controversy over the impact on bone density of increasing calcium consumption after menopause.

There is no indication that increasing calcium consumption in the *early* post-menopausal years will impact bone density. But a study by Bess Dawson-Hughes et al., compared changes in the bone mineral density of *late* postmenopausal women (had final menstrual period more than six years prior to the study), who consumed less than 400 mg/day of calcium, with a group of late postmenopausal women who consumed 400 to 650 mg/day. The results of the study showed that "Among the women who had been postmenopausal for six years or more...bone loss was less rapid in the group with the higher dietary calcium intake." [13]

The Dawson-Hughes study also showed that those late postmenopausal women who were consuming less than 400 mg/day of calcium could "...significantly reduce bone loss by increasing their calcium intake to 800 mg per day." This can be done through diet or supplementation. In the Dawson-Hughes study, *calcium citrate malate* was shown to be a more effective supplement than calcium carbonate.

There is no conclusive evidence as yet that post-menopausal women's bones can benefit from increasing calcium consumption to 1500 mg/day, as has been recommended by health organizations and dairy associations in North America.

In fact, a comparison of hip fracture rates to calcium consumption levels in different countries showed some of the lowest hip fracture rates in countries where calcium consumption in the general population is the lowest (e.g., 600 mg/day or less in Papua New Guinea, Hong Kong, Singapore, Yugoslavia), and some of the highest hip fracture rates in countries where calcium consumption in the general population is highest (e.g., greater than 900 mg/day in New Zealand, Norway, Sweden, Denmark, U.K., U.S.). [14]

Results of an often cited study of Alaskan Eskimos [15], reinforce the point that consuming large amounts of calcium after the bone formation years (i.e., after about 30 years of age) will not necessarily save your bones.

In that study, the Eskimo women were found to have bone mineral content similar to their U.S. white counterparts during the bone formation years, but after that their rate of bone mineral loss appeared to approximate 3% to 6% per decade *greater than* that of the corresponding whites, so that by the time the Eskimo women were in their 70s, they had a "...deficit of bone with respect to white values...[of] almost 30% below [comparable white values]." That is, the Eskimo women in their 70s had 30% less bone mineral content than their white counterparts.

The Eskimo women's low bone mineral content levels were in spite of daily calcium consumption in the range of 500-2500 mg, compared with what is widely regarded as being the norm for North American women of 400-500 mg/day. The Eskimos were also found not to be deficient in Vitamin D or lacking in exercise. The factor thought most likely to cause the high bone loss was the Eskimos' high meat diet. The next section will expand on this point.

Consumption of Foods of Animal Origin

A diet high in *non-dairy* foods of animal origin (i.e., meat, fish, fowl, eggs) is now being considered as possibly one of the primary causes of osteoporosis because of the acid-producing, bone-leaching nature of the protein found in these foods. (There is controversy over whether dairy products fit into this category.)

As the amount of non-dairy animal protein in the diet increases, excretion of calcium through the urine has been shown to increase. As the amount of protein from plant sources increases, excretion of calcium through the urine has been shown to decrease. [16]

Studies have linked diets high in non-dairy foods of animal origin to lower bone densities in older populations. Going back to the Eskimo study referred to above, animal protein consumption in the Eskimos in that study approximated 200-400 grams a day. This is 10 times the nutritionally required amount, and 2-4 times that of their U.S. white counterparts.

The previously mentioned study that compared hip fracture rates to calcium consumption in different countries, also compared hip fracture rates to animal protein consumption in those same countries.

That study found some of the highest hip fracture rates in countries where animal protein consumption in the general population was highest (e.g., greater than 55 gms/day in New Zealand, Norway, Sweden, Denmark, U.K., U.S. whites), and some of the lowest hip fracture rates in countries where animal protein consumption in the general population was lowest (e.g., 35 gms/day or less in Papua New Guinea, Hong Kong, Singapore, Yugoslavia). Note that these are the same countries with the highest and lowest calcium consumption, respectively. [17]

Low consumption of animal protein is considered to protect bone mass. Studies have shown lacto-ovo-vegetarians (consume dairy products and eggs but no other foods of animal origin) to experience a much lower incidence of bone loss in the later years than meat-eaters. [18-20]

In one large study, bone mineral mass of lacto-ovo-vegetarian women did not differ significantly from that of meat-eaters, up to about age 50. Then, between the ages of 50 and 89, meat-eating women lost *35%* of bone mineral mass as compared to *18%* for lacto-ovo-vegetarians. [21] This could be the difference between moving well into the "theoretical fracture zone" (and being classified as osteoporotic) and staying above it.

Physical Activity

Regular, moderate, aerobic, weight-bearing exercise can *prevent bone loss and increase bone mass and strength after menopause.* Weight-bearing exercise has been shown to add bone mass at any age, even in the eighties and nineties. Positive results are experienced in a short time, but are reversed if exercise is stopped. [22-24]

Regular physical activity also maintains or improves balance and co-ordination, thereby reducing the risk of falling. Since "... approximately 90 percent of hip fractures in the elderly result from a simple fall..." [25], reducing the risk of falling is another good reason to exercise regularly.

30 minutes a day, or 1 hour three times a week, can be effective in preventing post-menopausal bone loss. In this case, *more is better.* Be as physically active as possible.

Vitamin D

Vitamin D boosts calcium absorption and can be obtained through diet or from sunlight. Vitamin D production is turned on in your system when sunshine touches your unprotected skin (i.e., no sunscreen).

Vitamin D is critical in its function of helping your body absorb calcium from foods. 15 minutes of direct or indirect sunlight 2-3 times a week is all it takes. If this is not possible, 400 mg/day in a Vitamin D supplement is recommended. (Be sure to restrict exposure to direct sunlight to early morning or late evening, when cancer-causing ultra-violet rays are at their lowest levels.)

Other Factors Considered to Increase Bone Loss

- Smoking
- Alcohol   (inhibits calcium absorption)
- Carbonated drinks   (high in phosphorous)
- Caffeine   (e.g., in tea, coffee, chocolate, colas)
- Sugar   (includes glucose, maple syrup, honey, fructose, rice syrup, barley malt, corn syrup, molasses, dextrose)

- Sodium/Salt   (used as a preservative in packaged, canned and bottled foods, cured meats, and snack foods)

- Steroids   (e.g., cortisone, prednisone)
- Antibiotics   (especially tetracyclines)
- Sedatives, diuretics
- Lupron
- High fat diet   (reduces calcium absorption)
- Oxalic acid   (found in chocolate, spinach, Swiss chard, parsley, beet greens & rhubarb)
- Aluminum   (found in beverage cans, cookware, tap water, some antacids)
- Hypothyroidism & thyroid drugs

Special Discussion about Dairy Products

There is uncertainty and disagreement among the "experts" as to whether or not dairy products are a beneficial source of calcium.

The debate centres around the type of protein found in dairy products. Is it the same acid-producing, bone-leaching protein found in all other foods of animal origin? Or is it an alkaline protein like that found in most plant foods?

Neither the National Osteoporosis Foundation in the U.S. nor the Osteoporosis Society of Canada makes a distinction between dairy proteins and other animal proteins. This leaves us on our own to decide what role dairy products should play in our personal bone protection program.

In view of the generally denser bones of lacto-ovo-vegetarians as compared with meat-eaters (as found in many previously referenced studies), there seems to be no harm in consuming calcium from dairy products, if other animal products (i.e., meat, fish, fowl) are eliminated or minimized in our diet.

MANAGE AND PROTECT YOUR BONE HEALTH STARTING RIGHT NOW

Taking all the above findings into consideration, the following is a recommended course of action for minimizing your risk of osteoporosis, without drugs.

1. Have a bone density test to determine your current bone density. Use the results as a baseline from which to monitor your bone health throughout the post-menopausal years. After that, have regular bone density tests, as recommended in Chapter 5.

2.   Consume at least 800 mg of calcium daily, primarily from leafy green vegetables, legumes (beans), whole grains, and some low-fat dairy (optional).

3.   Minimize or eliminate from your diet, non-dairy foods of animal origin (i.e., meat, fish, fowl).

4.   Keep overall protein consumption down to your daily requirement.

5.   Increase regular, moderate, aerobic, weight-bearing exercise. Try to exercise for at least 30 minutes a day, or 1 hour three times a week. Be as physically active as possible.

6.   Enjoy 15 minutes of direct or indirect sunlight 2-3 times a week to obtain essential Vitamin D. Take 400 mg/day Vitamin D supplement, if sunlight exposure is not possible.

7.   Eliminate from your lifestyle as many as possible of the "Other Factors Considered to Increase Bone Loss" identified earlier in this chapter.

References

1. Peck, W.A., Burckhardt, P., Christiansen, C., et al. "Consensus Development Conference: Diagnosis, Prophylaxis, and Treatment of Osteoporosis." *American Journal of Medicine* 1993; 94:646-650.
2. Kanis, J. A., Melton, L. J. III, Christiansen, C., Johnston, C. C., and Khaltaev, N. "Perspective : The Diagnosis of Osteoporosis." *Journal of Bone and Mineral Research* 1994; 9 (8): 1137-1141.
3. Greenspan, S. L., Myers, E. R., Maitland, L. A., Resnick, N. M., and Hayes, W. C. "Fall severity and bone mineral density as risk factors for hip fracture in ambulatory elderly." *Journal of American Medical Association* 1994; 271:128-133.
4. Slemenda, C. W. and Johnston, C. C. Jr. "Epidemiology of Osteoporosis." In *Treatment of the Postmenopausal Woman: Basic and Clinical Aspects*, Lobo, R. A. (ed.). New York: Raven Press, Ltd., 1994, pp. 161-168.
5. Heaney, R. P. and Matkovic, V. "Inadequate Peak Bone Mass." In *Osteoporosis: Etiology, Diagnosis, and Management*, Riggs, B. L. and Melton, L. J. III (eds.). 2nd Edition, Philadelphia: Lippincott-Raven, 1995, p. 115.
6. Lindsay, R. "Estrogen Deficiency." In *Osteoporosis: Etiology, Diagnosis, and Management*, Riggs, B. L. and Melton, L. J. III (eds.). 2nd Edition, Philadelphia: Lippincott-Raven, 1995, p. 134.
7. Pouilles, J. M., Tremollieres, F., and Ribot, C. "The Effects of Menopause on Longitudinal Bone Loss from the Spine." *Calcified Tissue International* 1993; 52: 340-343.
8. Riggs, B. L., Wahner, H., Melton, L. J. III, Richelson, L. S., Judd, H. L., Offord, K. P. "Rates of bone loss in the appendicular and axial skeletons of women. Evidence of substantial vertebral bone loss before menopause." *Journal of Clinical Investigation* 1986; 77: 1487-1491.
9. Krolner, B., Pors Nielson, S. "Bone mineral content of the lumbar spine in normal and osteoporotic women: cross-sectional and longitudinal studies." *Clinical Science* 1982; 62: 329-336.
10. Nilas, L. and Christiansen, C. "Rates of bone loss in normal women: evidence of accelerated trabecular bone loss after the menopause." *European Journal of Clinical Investigation* 1988; 18: 529-534.
11. Harris, S. and Dawson-Hughes, B. "Rates of change in bone mineral density of spine, heel, femoral neck and radius in healthy postmenopausal women." *Bone and Mineral* 1992; 17: 87-95.
12. Bullamore, J. R., Gallagher, J. C., Wilkinson, R., Nordin, B. E. C., Marshall, D. H. "Effect of age on calcium absorption." *Lancet* 1970; 2: 535-537.
13. Dawson-Hughes, B., et al. "A Controlled Trial of the Effect of Calcium Supplementation on Bone Density in Postmenopausal Women." *The New England Journal of Medicine* 1990; 323 (13): 878-883.
14. Abelow, B. J., Holford, T. R., Insogna, K. L. "Cross-Cultural Association Between Dietary Animal Protein and Hip Fracture: A Hypothesis." *Calcified Tissue International* 1992; 50: 14-18.
15. Mazess, R. B. and Mather, W. "Bone Mineral Content of North Alaskan Eskimos." *American Journal of Clinical Nutrition* 1974; 27: 916-925.

16. Hu, J-F., Zhao, X-H., Parpia, B., and Campbell, T.C. "Dietary intakes and urinary excretion of calcium and acids: a cross-sectional study of women in China." *American Journal of Clinical Nutrition* 1993; 58: 398-406.

17. Abelow, B. J., Holford, T. R., Insogna, K. L. "Cross-Cultural Association Between Dietary Animal Protein and Hip Fracture: A Hypothesis." *Calcified Tissue International* 1992; 50: 14-18.

18. Ellis, F. R. , Holesh, S., and Ellis, J. W. "Incidence of Osteoporosis in Vegetarians and Omnivores." *American Journal of Clinical Nutrition* 1972; 25:555-558.

19. Sanchez, T. V., Mickelsen, O., Marsh, A. G., Garn, S. M., and Mayor, G. H. "Bone Mineral in Elderly Vegetarian and Omnivorous Females." In: Mazess R. B. ed. *Proceedings of the fourth international conference on bone measurement.* Bethesda, MD: NIAMMD 1980:94-8 (NIH publication #80-1983.)

20. Marsh, A. G., Sanchez, T. V., Mickelsen, O., Keiser, J., and Mayor, G. "Cortical Bone Density of Adult Lacto-Ovo-Vegetarian and Omnivorous Women." *Journal of American Dietetic Association* 1980; 76: 148-151.

21. Marsh, A. G., Sanchez, T. V., Mickelsen, O., Chaffee, F. L., and Fagal, S. M. "Vegetarian Lifestyle and Bone Mineral Density." *American Journal of Clinical Nutrition* 1988; 48: 837-841.

22. Dalsky, G. P., Stocke, K. S., Ehsani, A. A., Slatopolsky, E., Lee, W. C., and Birge, S. J. "Weight-Bearing Exercise Training and Lumbar Bone Mineral Content in Postmenopausal Women." *Annals of Internal Medicine* 1988; 108: 824-828.

23. Rikli, R. R. and McManis, B. G. "Effects of Exercise on Bone Mineral Content in Postmenopausal Women." *Research Quarterly for Exercise and Sport* 1990; 61: 243-249.

24. Chow, R., Harrison, J. E., and Notarius, C. "Effect of Two Randomised Exercise Programmes on Bone Mass of Healthy Postmenopausal Women." *British Medical Journal* 1987; 295: 1441-1444.

25. Zuckerman, J. D. "Hip Fracture." *The New England Journal of Medicine* 1996; 334 (23): 1519-1525.

10
SEVEN-STEP PROGRAM SUMMARY

This *seven-step program* has been designed to guide and support you through your menopausal years, and to help you establish a plan to make the next stage of your life a longer, healthier one. The steps are recapped below.

STEP 1: *Set Up a Menopause Tracking System.*

Start tracking your symptoms and your menstrual periods as part of an information gathering exercise. This will help to:

- Confirm that you *are* going through menopause

- Reduce fear and uncertainty about the cause of symptoms

- Focus appropriate treatment on the underlying cause of the symptoms

STEP 2: *Find a Health Practitioner You Trust.*

A good health practitioner can mean the difference between a difficult menopausal experience and a more manageable one. It is important to have a knowledgeable, supportive health practitioner as a partner for this time in your life and beyond.

STEP 3: *Complete the Process of Medical Testing.*

Tests can help to identify underlying causes of symptoms and provide early warnings of potential future health problems. Medical tests are necessary to:

- Make sure that your symptoms are those of menopause and not an illness

- Keep on top of menopausal symptoms which can lead to serious health problems if left untreated

- Identify your body's areas of potential future weakness, so that you can take action now to improve your long-term health prospects, without drugs

STEP 4: *Identify Your Health Vulnerabilities.*

Test results can identify current and potential areas of weakness in your health, if any. Awareness of such weaknesses, sooner rather than later, increases your chances of being able to minimize or eliminate them through gentle, non-drug methods.

STEP 5: *Relieve Menopausal Symptoms without Drugs.*

Try non-drug therapies for menopausal symptoms, first. They may be all you need to make it gently and safely through your menopausal years. Commonly used remedies are:

- Herbs
- Traditional Chinese Medicine
- Diet
- Exercise

STEP 6: *Start the Process of Changing to a Healthier Diet.*

The foods you eat play an enormous role in determining your health and the illnesses from which you will suffer in your lifetime. High consumption of foods of animal origin and fats are now considered to be major culprits in the development of human disease.

A diet is recommended which draws nutrients primarily from:

- Whole grains
- Legumes
- Fresh vegetables
- Fresh fruit
- Some low-fat dairy (optional)

and is low in:

- Fats
- Cholesterol

STEP 7: *Enjoy the Benefits of <u>Moderate</u> Exercise.*

Regular, *moderate*, aerobic, weight-bearing exercise provides physical, emotional, and intellectual health benefits.

30 minutes a day, or 1 hour three times a week, is sufficient for major health benefits. Find an exercise you enjoy and incorporate it into your day. Be as physically active as possible. In this case, *more is better.*

Take your time. Make the effort.
It is important to your health and to your future.

SELECTED BIBLIOGRAPHY OF BOOKS

Appleton, Nancy. *Healthy Bones*. New York: Avery Publishing Group Inc., 1991.

Barbach, Lonnie. *The Pause: Positive Approaches to Menopause*. New York: Signet/Penguin, 1994.

Barnard, Neal. *Eat Right, Live Longer*. New York: Harmony Books, 1995.

Chen, J., Campbell, T. C., Li J., Peto, R. *Diet, Life-style and Mortality in China: A Study of the Characteristics of 65 Chinese Counties*. Oxford: Oxford University Press, 1990.

Cobb, Janine O'Leary. *Understanding Menopause*. Toronto: Key Porter Books, 1993.

Coney, Sandra. *The Menopause Industry*. Alameda, California: Hunter House Inc., 1994.

Dunne, Lavon J. *Nutrition Almanac*. New York: McGraw-Hill, 1990.

Eades, Mary Dan. *The Doctor's Complete Guide to Vitamins and Minerals*. New York: Dell Publishing, 1994.

Fox, Arnold and Fox, Barry. *Immune for Life*. Rocklin, California: Prima Publishing, 1989.

Furman, C. Sue. *Turning Point*. New York: Oxford University Press, 1995.

Greenwood, Sadja. *Menopause Naturally*. Volcano, CA: Volcano Press, 1989.

Griffith, H. Winter. *Complete Guide to Symptoms, Illness & Surgery*. Los Angeles: Body Press, 1989.

Griffith, H. Winter. *Complete Guide to Prescription & Non-Prescription Drugs*. New York: The Berkley Publishing Group, 1997.

Health and Welfare Canada. *Nutrient Value of Some Common Foods*. Ottawa, Canada: Canadian Government Publishing Centre for Supply and Services Canada, 1988.

Jovanovic, Lois with LeVert, Suzanne. *A Woman Doctor's Guide to Menopause*. New York: Hyperion, 1993.

Lark, Susan M. *The Menopause Self Help Book*. Berkeley, California: Celestial Arts, 1990.

Lee, John R. *What Your Doctor May Not Tell You About Menopause*. New York: Warner Books, Inc, 1996.

Love, Susan. *Dr. Susan Love's Breast Book*. 2nd Edition. Reading, Massachusetts: Addison-Wesley, 1995.

Love, Susan. *Dr. Susan Love's Hormone Book*. New York: Random House, 1997.

Maas, Paula, Brown, Susan E. and Bruning, Nancy. *Natural Medicine for Menopause and Beyond*. New York: Dell Publishing, 1997.

McDougall, John A. *The McDougall Program for a Healthy Heart*. New York: Dutton/Penguin, 1996.

Mindell, Earl. *Earl Mindell's Vitamin Book*. New York: Warner Books, 1991.

Mindell, Earl. *Earl Mindell's Food as Medicine*. New York: Fireside/Simon & Schuster, 1994.

Mindell, Earl. *Earl Mindell's Soy Miracle*. New York: Fireside/Simon & Schuster, 1995.

Netzer, Corinne T. *The Corinne T. Netzer Vitamin and Mineral Counter*. New York: Dell Publishing, 1996.

Ojeda, Linda. *Menopause Without Medicine*. Alameda, CA: Hunter House Inc., 1992.

Ornish, Dean, *Dr. Dean Ornish's Program for Reversing Heart Disease*. New York: Ivy Books, 1996.

Polunin, Miriam. *The Knopf Canada Book of Healing Foods*. Toronto: Alfred A. Knopf Canada, 1997.

Reid, Daniel P. *Chinese Herbal Medicine*. Boston: Shambhala Publications, Inc., 1986.

Riggs, B.L. and Melton, L.J. (eds.). *Osteoporosis: Etiology, Diagnosis, and Management*. 2nd Edition. Philadelphia, Pennsylvania: Lippincott-Raven Publishers, 1995.

Ring, E.F.J., Elvins, D.M. and Bhalla, A.K. (eds.). *Current Research in Osteoporosis and Bone Mineral Measurement IV: 1996*. London, England: British Institute of Radiology, 1996.

Sheehy, Gail. *The Silent Passage*. New York: Random House, 1992.

Silverman, Harold M., Romano, Joseph A. and Elmer, Gary. *The Vitamin Book*. New York: Bantam Books, 1985.

Simkin, Ariel and Ayalon, Judith. *Bone Loading*. London, England: Prion, 1990.

Somer, Elizabeth. *The Essential Guide to Vitamins and Minerals*. New York: Harper Collins, 1992.

Stoppard, Miriam. *Menopause*. Toronto: Random House of Canada, 1994.

Ulene, Art. *The NutriBase Guide to Fat & Cholesterol in Your Food*. New York: Avery Publishing Group, 1995.

Weed, Susun S. *Menopausal Years: The Wise Woman Way*. Woodstock, New York: Ash Tree Publishing, 1992.

INDEX

Ablation. *See* Endometrial ablation

Acne (HRT side-effect), 24

Acupuncture/acupressure, 71
  for depression, 79
  for heavy bleeding, 74
  for hot flashes/night sweats, 77
  for mental acuity, 80

Addiction, drug, 22

Additives, food, 94

Adrenal glands
  function test, 43

Aging, 11
  and calcium, 102

Alcohol, 72, 76, 79, 80, 115

Allergy-causing substances, 90

Alternative therapies, 68-74.
  See also Chinese medicine; Diet;
  Exercise; Herbs; Naturopathy

Aluminum
  and bone loss, 116

Amino acids, 94

Anemia blood tests
  for heavy bleeding, 74

Anemia, iron-deficiency, 12, 13, 36
  from heavy bleeding, 11, 75-76
  hemoglobin/ferritin level test, 43

Angelica sinensis. *See* Dong quai

Antibiotics, 15
  and bone loss, 116

Anti-depressants, 23.
  See also Elavil; Prozac

Anti-oxidants, 97-100

Anxiety, 12, 17, 79
  drug side-effect, 23

Dong quai for, 70
  exercise and, 73
  as hyperthyroidism symptom, 36
  non-drug suggestions for, 79-80
  use of herbs to treat, 69

Appetite changes (HRT side-effect), 24

Arthritis. *See* Menopause arthritis

Aspirin
  iron depletion from, 76

Backache, 16, 23

Bacterial infections, 15

Behaviour changes (drug side-effect), 22

Beta-carotene
  anti-oxidant properties of, 97.
  See also Vitamin A

Bioflavonoids, 72, 73, 78
  for anxiety, 79
  for heavy bleeding, 74
  for hot flashes/night sweats, 77
  to lessen depression, 79
  supplements, 98

Birth defects, 6

Black cohosh
  for hot flashes/night sweats, 77

Bladder infections.
  See Urinary tract infections

Bladder tests, 43

Bleeding, heavy/flooding
  acupuncture/acupressure for, 71, 74
  anemia from, 11, 75-76
  bioflavonoids for, 74
  Chinese medicine for, 75
  Dong quai for, 70

foods offering relief from, 71-72
hysterectomies and, 74
naturopathy for, 75
non-drug suggestions for, 74-75
progesterone for, 75
tests for, 74.
See also Endometrial ablation
Blood clotting (HRT side-effect), 24
Blood discharge, 5
Blood pressure, high, 55
lowering of through exercise, 105
lowering of through Vitamin E, 98
BMD, 57, 59-60
and age ranges, 61
Bone density, 111-112
and calcium consumption, 102, 113-114
exercise and, 105, 107
and HRT, 24
loss of, 44, 112, 113, 115-116
maintaining bone health (checklist), 116-117
protecting bone mass, 62-63, 115
and Vitamin A intake, 99
Bone density tests, 36, 40
checklist, 45
data in, 59-60
frequency, 40
graphs of, 60-62, 112
recommended, 116
reviewing, 57-62
Bone fracture(s)
causes of, 63
HRT and, 63
risk of, 58, 62-63
Bone mineral density.
See BMD
Bone pain, 12
Bowel function, 43
Breast tenderness, 12, 16
HRT side-effect, 24
using Evening Primrose oil
to relieve, 73

Breasts, tests of, 40-42
checklist, 45
frequency, 41
mammograms, 40-41
physical exam, 41
self-examination (BSE), 42, 47-48
(illustrated)
Breathing difficulty, 12

Caffeine, 10, 72, 76, 77, 79, 94, 115
Calcium
absorption of through Vitamin D, 115
and bone loss, 113
dairy products as source of, 102-103, 116
food sources of (tables), 103-104
function of, 102
and hip fractures, 113, 114
increased consumption of, 102-104, 113-114, 117
supplements, 104, 113
Calories
from fat intake, 87
Cancer, 83
breast, 24, 97
colon, 43, 97
diet and, 84, 86
exercise and, 105
fibre for reduced risk of, 100
ovarian, 36, 97
uterine, 24
vitamins and, 98, 99
Carbohydrates, 88
Carbonated drinks, 76, 115
Cardiovascular disease
and cholesterol level, 92
diet and, 84, 86
exercise and, 105
fibre for reduced risk of, 100
genetic history and, 85
HRT and, 24, 25, 93
post-menopausal, 83
reducing risks of, 21, 25, 83

reversal diet (Ornish), 87
and vitamins, 98, 99
Cardiovascular medical tests, 36, 39-40
checklist, 45
frequency, 40
reviewing, 54-57
Castelli, Dr. William, 57, 93
Chemotherapy, 8
Childbirth, child-raising, 6
Chills (drug side-effect), 22
Chinese medicine, traditional, 12, 69-71
for heavy bleeding, 75
Cholesterol
levels of, 56-57, 92-94
manufacture of in body, 88
misleading claims about, 93
in North American vs. Chinese diets, 56
total, defined, 55
understanding, 55-56
and Vitamin E, 98
Climacteric, 3.
See also Menopausal symptoms; Menopause
Colitis, 43
Colon, medical tests of, 43
Concentration loss, 15, 19
as anemia symptom, 75-76
Dong quai for, 70-71
non-drug suggestions for, 80
Confusion
as anemia symptom, 75-76
drug side-effect, 22
Constipation
drug side-effect, 22, 23
fibre intake for reducing, 100
Counselling, 78
Cramping, 13, 16
drug side-effect, 23
HRT side-effect, 24
Crying. *See* Weepiness
Cysts
cancerous, 36

HRT side-effect, 24
ovarian, 17, 36

Dairy products, 71, 78, 85, 86, 116
as calcium source, 102-103
fat content of, 88
iron depletion from, 76.
See also Protein, animal-origin
Dandelion
for depression, 79
as iron source, 76
Dang gui.
See Dong quai
Decision-making difficulties, 19, 80
Depression/sadness, 12, 17, 44, 78-79
drug side-effect, 22
Dong quai for, 70-71
exercise and, 73
foods offering relief from, 71-72
hormonally vs. psychologically induced, 8
HRT benefit (relieves), 23
HRT side-effect, 24
non-drug suggestions for, 78-79
Diabetes
exercise and, 105
medical tests for, 44
Diarrhea, 13, 14
drug side-effect, 22, 23
HRT side-effect, 24
Diet, 10
and bone loss, 116
changing to a healthier (Step 6), 84-104, 122
hot flashes/night sweats and, 76-77
intellectual/emotional symptoms and, 78
low-fat, 85
North American, 83
recommended, 71-72, 84
vegetarian, 84, 95, 98, 103, 115, 116
Digestive upset, 14
acupuncture/acupressure for, 71

Diverticulosis, 100
Dizziness/lightheadedness, 12, 13, 15, 18
  as anemia symptom, 75-76
  drug side-effect, 22
  HRT benefit (relieves), 23
  HRT side-effect, 24
Dong quai, 12, 52, 70-71
  for anxiety, 79
  for depression, 79
  for hot flashes/night sweats, 77
  for mental acuity, 80
Dowager's hump, 58
Drowsiness (drug side-effect), 22, 23
Drugs, 21, 26
  alternatives to, 26
  and bone loss, 116
  side-effects of, 1, 12, 21-23
  types of, 22-23. *See also* Chinese
  medicine; Herbal treatments; HRT;
  specific medications; tranquilizers
Dry mouth/burning sensation, 16

Elavil, 23
Electrocardiogram, 57
Eleutherococcus. *See* Siberian ginseng
Endometrial ablation, 75
Endometrial biopsy, 42
Estraderm, 23
Estrogen, estrogen levels, 4
  charting, 52-54
  effect of on body, 8
  imbalance of with progesterone, 4-5, 8
  as menopause indicator, 50-54
  plant sources of, 70
  in post-menopausal years, 5, 6-7
  pre-pubertal, 6
  primary source of, 8
  purpose of, 83
  side-effects of (HRT), 24
  surges in, 36.
  See also HRT; Phytoestrogens
Evening Primrose oil, 73, 77

Exercise, 73-74
  aerobic, 104-105
  cautions involving, 107
  enjoying benefits of moderate (Step 7),
  10, 78, 84, 104-108, 117, 122
  for hot flashes/night sweats, 77
  and increased bone mass, 115
  weight-bearing, 104-105

Faintness (HRT side-effect), 24
Fat(s)
  calories in, 88
  consumption, 10, 87-92, 94
  content of food groups, 88
  misleading claims about, 91-92
  requirements, 89-91
  types of, 88-89, 93, 94
Fatigue, 13, 14, 44
  as anemia symptom, 75-76
  as diabetes symptom, 36
  drug side-effect, 23
  exercise and, 73, 106
  herbs for, 69
  HRT side-effect, 24
  as hyperthyroidism symptom, 36
  non-drug suggestions for, 75-76
Fearfulness, 18
Feet, swollen (HRT side-effect), 24
Fever
  drug side-effect, 22
  HRT side-effect, 24
Fibre
  food sources of (table), 101
  function of, 100
  recommended intake of, 100-101
Fibroids, 17
  growth in, 36
  HRT side-effect, 24
Fish
  fat content of, 88
Flashes, hot. *See* Hot flashes
Floradix Formula Herbal Iron Extract, 76
Follicle-stimulating hormone. *See* FSH

Food(s)
  avoiding specific, 72
  iron-depleting/iron rich, 76
  recommended daily consumption (chart), 86
  as source of bioflavonoids, 72.
  See also Diet
Fractures. *See* Bone fracture(s)
Free-radicals, 97, 98
Fruit, fresh, 71, 72, 77, 78, 85, 86, 94, 97
  and calcium, 95
  fat content of, 88
  fibre content of, 101
FSH (follicle-stimulating hormone)
  levels, 38, 50-52

Gallstone risk (HRT side-effect), 24
Ginseng, Siberian
  for depression, 79
Grains, whole, 71, 72, 77, 78, 85, 86, 94, 97
  fat content of, 88
  fibre content of, 101

Hallucinations (drug side-effect), 22, 23
HDL, 55
  ratio, 56-57, 93-94
Headache, 12, 15
  Dong quai for, 70
  drug side-effect, 22, 23
  HRT side-effect, 24
Head shocks, 15
Health practitioner, trusted
  finding (Step 2), 121
  qualities of, 35
Health vulnerabilities
  identifying (Step 4), 49-65, 122
Hearing disorders, 12, 16
Heart attack
  risk of, 56, 57
Heartbeat, irregular/rapid
  as anemia symptom, 75-76
  drug side-effect, 23

Heart disease.
  See Cardiovascular disease
Heart palpitations, 15
  Dong quai for, 70
  drug side-effect, 23
  HRT benefit (relieves), 23
Heavy bleeding/flooding.
  See Bleeding
Hemorrhoids, 43, 100
Herbs, herbal treatments, 68-69
  for anxiety, 79
  cautions for use of, 68-69
  Chinese, 70-71
  for depression, 79
  for hot flashes/night sweats, 77
  iron-rich, 76
  for mental acuity, 80.
  See also Dong quai
High blood pressure, 87
High-density lipoprotein. *See* HDL
Hip fracture(s), 58
  and calcium consumption, 114
Hives (HRT side-effect), 24
Hologic report (bone densitometry), 58-62
Hormone(s)
  blood tests, 50-51
  changes and imbalances, 1, 8, 9, 10
  levels, 83
  ovarian, 112-113
  receptors, 8
  tracking system, 51-54. *See also* Estrogen; Progestin
Hormone Replacement Therapy.
  See HRT
Hot flashes/night sweats, 12, 13, 15, 18, 44, 77
  acupuncture/acupressure for, 71
  Dong quai for, 70
  drug side-effect 23
  Evening Primrose oil for, 73
  exercise and, 73, 106
  foods offering relief from, 71-72

HRT benefit (relieves), 23
  non-drug suggestions for, 76-77
  Vitamin E to relieve, 73
HRT, 23-25
  benefits of, immediate, 23-24
  benefits of, prolonged use, 24
  and bone-density loss, 24
  and bone fracture, 63
  calcium consumption and, 102
  and cardiovascular protection, 24, 25, 93
  drug forms of, 23
  genetic history and, 85
  and intellectual and emotional
  symptoms, 77
  and osteoporosis, 25, 63
  risks from, 24-25, 67
  side-effects of, 24, 67, 84.
  See also Estraderm, Premarin, Provera
Hyperplasia, 36
Hypertension. *See* Blood pressure, high
Hyperthyroidism/hypothyroidism
  climacteric-like symptoms of, 44
  thyroid function tests, 44
Hyperventilation, 14
Hysterectomy, 8, 9, 10, 74

Indigestion (drug side-effect), 23
Infections
  and antibiotics, 15.
  See also Bacterial, Intestinal, Yeast
  infections
Insomnia. *See* Sleep disorders
Intellectual function impairment
  (drug side-effect), 22
Intercourse, painful, 15, 17, 36
Intestinal infection, 43
Iron-deficiency anemia. *See* Anemia
Iron supplements, 76
Irritability, 18
  drug side-effect, 22
  foods offering relief from, 71-72
  HRT benefit (relieves), 23
  HRT side-effect, 24

Itchiness, 12, 15, 16
  HRT side-effect, 24

Jaundice (HRT side-effect), 24
Joint pain, soreness
  exercise and, 73, 106
  herbs for treating, 69

Kidney medical tests, 43

LDL, 55
Legumes, 10, 71, 72, 77, 78, 85, 86
  fat content of, 88
  fibre content of, 101
Lethargy, 12
LH (luteinizing hormone)
  levels of, 37-38, 50-52
Liver
  function impairment (drug side-
  effect), 22
  function test, 43
Lorazepam, 22
Love, Dr. Susan, 25, 40, 41
Low-density lipoprotein. *See* LDL
Lunar report (bone densitometry), 58-62
Lupron
  adverse reactions to, 11-12
  and bone loss, 116
  symptoms caused by, 8

Mammograms, 40-41
McDougall, Dr. John, 54, 56, 57, 90, 93
Meat
  fat content of, 88.
  See also Protein, animal-origin
Medical tests, medical testing (general)
  checklists, 36, 37, 44, 45-46
  completing the process of (Step 3),
  35-48, 121
  for determining menopause, 50-54
  and hormone levels, 38-39
  and osteoporosis, 36
  preparing for, 36, 37-44

reasons for, 36
reviewing, 49-63.
See also specific tests: Bone density;
Breasts; Cardiovascular; Menopause-
related; Reproductive organs
Medical treatments
and difficult symptoms, 10
and menopausal symptoms, 9.
See also Chemotherapy;
Hysterectomy; Medical tests;
Radiation
Medication. *See* Drugs
Memory loss, 15, 19, 44
Dong quai for, 70-71
non-drug suggestions for, 80
Menopausal symptoms (general), 3, 6-7
duration of, 67
effect of on performance, 9
emotional, 17-18, 77-80
estrogen's role in, 6
foods offering relief from, 71-72
intellectual, 18-19, 77-80
physical, 12-17, 74-77
progesterone's role in, 6
relieving without drugs (Step 5),
67-81, 122
unnoticeable, 9
virus-like, 12, 13, 14
and Vitamin E, 98
vs. other symptoms, 11.
See also Diet; Drug side-effects;
Exercise; HRT side-effects; and
specific symptoms: Anxiety, Backache,
Bleeding, Bone pain, Breast
tenderness, Breathing difficulty,
Concentration loss, Decision-making,
Depression, Diarrhea, Digestive,
Dizziness, Dry mouth, Fatigue,
Fearfulness, Fibroids, Headache,
Hearing disorders, Heart palpitations,
Hot flashes/night sweats, Intercourse
(painful), Irritability, Itching, Joint
pain, Lethargy, Memory loss,
Menopause arthritis, Mental acuity
(reduced), Mood swings,
Nausea/vomiting, Nervousness,
Numbness, Ovarian cysts, Pain, Panic
attacks, PMS, Sensory disturbances,
Skin sensitivity, Sleep disorders,
Urinary tract, Urination,
Vision/ophthalmologic, Weakness,
Weepiness, Weight gain
Menopause, 3
climacteric process, 4-5
effects of, 8-10
indicators of, 37
reasons for occurrence of, 6
"unnatural" occurrences of, 7-8
years of, 7
Menopause arthritis, 16
Dong quai for, 70
Menopause-related medical tests 37-39
blood tests, 38-39
checklist, 45
frequency, 39
FSH and LH levels, 37-39
limitations of, 38
preparing for, 39
reviewing, 50-54
saliva testing technique, 39
Menopause tracking system
setting up (Step 1), 29-33, 121
Menstrual cycle(s)
calendar (sample), 31
chart (sample), 32-33
climacteric (illustrated), 5
menstruation changes (HRT side-
effect), 24
phases of, 51
pre-climacteric, 4
tracking, 29-30
varying lengths of, 5
Menstrual period(s)
changing patterns of, 12-13
disorders, 44
Dong quai for irregular, 70

final, 3, 4
missed, 36
painful (drug side-effect) 23
Mental acuity, reduced, 19, 44
Milk
calories and fat content in, 91
Mood swings, 12, 18
acupuncture/acupressure relief for, 71
foods offering relief from, 71-72
HRT benefit (relieves), 23
Mouth, dry (drug side-effect) 22, 23
Muscles, 16

Nasal congestion (drug side-effect), 23
Naturopathy, 68
for heavy bleeding, 75
Nausea/vomiting, 13, 14, 18
drug side-effect, 22, 23
HRT side-effect, 24
Nervousness, 12, 17
drug side-effect, 23
Nightmares (drug side-effect), 23
Night sweats.
See Hot flashes/night sweats
Numbness, 12
HRT benefit (relieves), 23
Nuts and seeds
as calcium source, 103
fat content of, 88

Obesity
fibre intake for reducing, 100
Oils
saturated fat content of, 89
Oophorectomy, 8
Ornish, Dr. Dean, 87, 90, 93, 107
Osteoporosis, 36, 83, 111-112
and animal-protein foods, 95, 114-15
and bone density test, 40, 60, 62
calcium's role in offsetting, 102
characteristics of, 95
diet and, 84, 86
genetic history and, 85

and HRT, 25, 63
minimizing risk of (checklist), 116-117
protecting against, 21, 25
risk of developing, 58, 83
and vegetarian diet, 95
Ovarian cysts, 17, 36
Ovarian hormones, 112-113
Ovaries, removal of. See Oophorectomy
Oxalic acid
and bone loss, 116

Pain
abdominal and side, 22, 23, 24
calf, 24
eye, 23
joint, 16, 69, 23, 73, 106
shoulder, wrist, hands, 16.
See also Backache, Headache,
Intercourse (painful)
Panic attacks, 13, 15, 18
Pap smear, 42
Pelvic exam, 42
Perimenopause, 3
Physician. See Health practitioner
Phytoestrogens (plant estrogens)
foods containing, 71-72
PMS
as menopause indicator, 10
Vitamin E for, 98
worsening of, 17
Post-menopause, 3
hormone levels (illustrated), 5
Post-partum difficulties
as menopause indicator, 10
Pregnancy, 6
hormone-associated, 10
Premarin, 23
Progesterone, progesterone levels, 4
charting, 52-54
drug form of (Progestin), 24
effect of on body, 8
and heavy bleeding, 75
imbalance of with estrogen, 4-5, 8

as menopause indicator, 50-54
plant sources of, 70
in post-menopausal years, 5
purpose of, 83
Progestin
side-effects of, 24
Protein, 94
acid- vs. alkaline-producing, 95
calories in, 88
consumption, 117
requirements, 95
sources of, 94, 96 (table)
Protein, animal-origin
and calcium loss, 95, 102
effect of on osteoporosis, 95, 114-115
foods, 10
reducing intake of, 94-97, 117.
See also Dairy products
Provera, 23
Prozac, 23
Psychological state
relationship of to menopausal
suffering, 10
Puberty, 9

Radiation, 8
Rash (HRT side-effect), 24
Reproductive organs, medical
tests of, 42
checklist, 45
endometrial biopsy, 42
frequency, 42
for heavy bleeding, 74
pap smear, 42
pelvic exam, 42
transvaginal ultrasound, 42
Restlessness
as hyperthyroidism symptom, 36

Self-image, 10, 17
Sensory disturbances, 16
Seven-Step Program, 1, 27, 121-122
Shortness of breath

as anemia symptom, 75-76
Siberian ginseng
for hot flashes/night sweats, 77
Skin sensitivity, 16
Sleep disorders/disturbances, 12, 13, 14, 44
acupuncture/acupressure for, 71
Dong quai for, 70
drug side-effect, 23
Evening Primrose oil for, 73
exercise and, 73, 106
HRT side-effect, 24
as hyperthyroidism symptom, 36
use of herbs to treat, 69
Smoking, 77, 83, 94, 115
Sodium
and bone loss, 116
Soy products, 10, 72, 77, 78
Spine, 58
Steroids
and bone loss, 116
Stinging nettle, 69
Stress, 7, 9, 10
and hot flashes/night sweats, 77
Stroke
and cholesterol level, 92
exercise and, 105
risk of, 56
Sugar, 94
and anxiety, depression, 79
and bone loss, 115
consumption, 10
and hot flashes/night sweats, 77
impact of on symptoms, 72
and mental acuity, 80
Sweats, night.
See Hot flashes/night sweats
Symptoms, menopausal.
See Menopausal symptoms

TCM. *See* Chinese medicine, traditional
Teeth, 99, 102
Testosterone, 9
Tests, medical. *See* Medical tests

Thyroid
  condition, 36
  drugs and bone loss, 116
  function tests, 44
Tranquilizers
  side-effects of, 22
  use of, 22.
  See also Lorazepam, Valium
Transvaginal ultrasound, 42
Tremor (drug side-effect), 23
Triglycerides, 57

Urinary tract problems, 12
  HRT benefit (relieves), 23
  use of herbs to treat, 69
Urination difficulties, 15
  drug side-effect, 22, 23
  frequent urination, 36
  HRT benefit (relieves stress
  incontinence), 23
  incontinence, 12
Uterus
  lining of, 36
  removal of (hysterectomy), 8, 9, 10, 74

Vaginal problems, 15
  HRT benefit (relieves dryness), 23
  HRT side-effect (discharge), 24
  Vitamin E to relieve, 73
Valium, 22
Vegetables, 71, 72, 77, 78, 85, 86, 94, 97
  and calcium, 95
  fat content of, 88
  fibre content of, 101
Vegetarian diet
  and bone density, 116
  and bone loss, 115
  and calcium intake, 103
  and osteoporosis, 95
  Vitamin E in, 98
Vision/ophthalmologic disorders, 12, 16
  contact lens intolerance, 24
  drug side-effect, 22 (changes),

23 (blurred vision)
  HRT side-effect, 24
  and Vitamin A, 99
Vitamin A (Beta-carotene)
  anti-oxidant properties of, 97
  functions, sources, dosages of, 99
Vitamin Bs
  for calcium absorption, 104
  for depression, 79
  for mental acuity, 80
Vitamin C
  anti-oxidant properties of, 97
  for anxiety, 79
  for depression, 79
  functions, sources, dosages of, 73, 97-98
  for hot flashes/night sweats, 77
  supplemental form of, 100
Vitamin D
  for calcium absorption, 104, 115
  suggested dosage, 117
Vitamin E, 94
  anti-oxidant properties of, 97
  benefits from, 93
  functions, sources, dosages of, 73, 98-99
  for hot flashes/night sweats, 77
  supplemental form of, 100
Vitamin and mineral supplements, 99-100
Vitex
  for hot flashes/night sweats, 77

Water retention, 14
  use of herbs to treat, 69
Weakness, 12
  as anemia symptom, 75-76
  drug side-effect, 23
Weepiness, 13, 14, 15, 18
Weight gain/changes, 17
  HRT side-effect, 24
Wheat sensitivity, 14
Wine, red
  and hot flashes/night sweats, 77

Yeast infections, 15

MAIL ORDER FORM

If you would like us to mail to you or a friend a copy of

A Seven-Step Program
for Getting Through
Menopause
and Enjoying a
Longer, Healthier Life
without drugs

Complete the information requested below and forward along with payment.

In Canada: $22.95 per copy in Cdn dollar cheque or money order

Outside Canada: $16.95 per copy in U.S. dollar cheque or money order

Payable To: ***Health Issues***

Address: P.O. Box 64, Station Q
                             Toronto, Canada
                             M4T 2L7

Number of copies requested _____ ✕ _____ = \$_____ enclosed
                                                                    (price)

Name_____
                                        (please print)

Address _____

Town/City _____   Province/State _____

Country _____   Postal/Zip Code_____

Telephone (   ) _____

(All applicable taxes, shipping and handling charges included.)